Obstetric Medicine

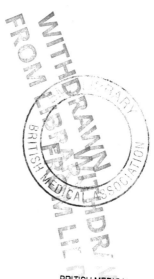

Obstetric Medicine

A Problem-Based Approach

Catherine Nelson-Piercy

and

Joanna Girling

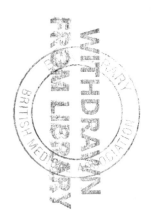

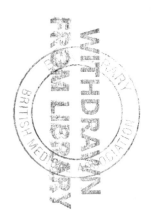

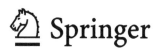 Springer

Catherine Nelson-Piercy, MA, FRCP
Consultant Obstetric Physician
Guy's & St Thomas' NHS Foundation Trust
Queen Charlotte's Hospital
London, UK

Joanna Girling, MA, MRCP, FRCOG
Consultant Obstetrician & Gynaecologist
West Middlesex University Hospital
Isleworth, UK

British Library Cataloguing in Publication Data
Nelson-Piercy, Catherine
    Maternal medicine in clinical practice
    1. Obstetrics - Examinations, questions, etc. 2. Obstetrics - Case studies
    I. Title II, Girling, Joanna
    618.2'0076

ISBN-10: 1-84628-563-1   e-ISBN-10: 1-84628-582-8
ISBN-13: 978-1-84628-563-9   e-ISBN-13: 978-1-84628-582-0

Printed on acid-free paper

9 8 7 6 5 4 3 2 1

Springer Science+Business Media
springer.com

Preface

Medical problems in pregnancy are common. They are responsible for much maternal and fetal morbidity and mortality. Recognition of the importance of maternal medicine is now reflected in the content of the membership exam of Royal College of Obstetricians and Gynaecologists (MRCOG), core training and higher training in both obstetrics and medicine.

Originally, this book was intended to be a collection of multiple choice questions, data interpretation and short answer questions, and model essay answers in obstetric medicine to help the trainee prepare for the MRCOG part 2. However, we appreciate that different trainees prepare and learn in different ways and that much practical maternal medicine is learnt after passing the MRCOG and membership exam of the Royal College of Physicians (MRCP). It was Tom Holland who had the idea to produce a collection of case studies to illustrate common problems in obstetric medicine and it was Ian Greer who had the idea to publish the case reports that trainees had written as part of their RCOG special skills module in maternal medicine. We are indebted to both.

So the finished product gives the trainee many different approaches to obstetric medicine. The extended matching questions require a large breadth of theoretical knowledge. The short answers and data interpretation require a systematic approach to a clinical problem. Most of the case reports, which range from esoteric to more mundane, are derived from real cases and all are accompanied by a brief literature review to further broaden the learning experience. Because the cases are real, the management described is not always perfect and is sometimes controversial. We have decided to leave in many of these unresolved issues to prompt the reader to think about, and read around, the topic. For this reason, key references used by the trainees in writing their case reports have been included. By contrast, the model essay answers provide a template of ideal management, as one would describe in an exam.

We hope that there is something for everyone and that trainees and, indeed, consultants will be able to "test themselves" using the different methods, in addition to reading about medical problems in pregnancy that they might not yet have encountered.

Catherine Nelson-Piercy
Consultant Obstetric Physician
Guy's & St Thomas' Hospital
Queen Charlotte's Hospital
London

Joanna Girling
Consultant Obstetrician & Gynaecologist
West Middlesex University Hospital
Isleworth

January 2007

Contents

Contributors to the Case Studies

Catherine Calderwood, MA CANTAB, MRCOG
Consultant Obstetrician and Gynaecologist
Simpson Centre for Reproductive Health
Royal Infirmary of Edinburgh *and*
St John's Hospital, Livingston, UK

Sonji D. Clarke, MBBS, MRCOG
Consultant Obstetrician and Gynaecologist
Guy's and St Thomas' Hospitals Foundation Trust
London, UK

Douglas P. Dumbrill, FCOG(SA), MRCOG
Consultant Obstetrician and Gynaecologist
112 Vincent Pallotti Medical Centre
Alexander Road
Pinelands 7405
Capetown, South Africa

Tom Holland, MBBS
Research Fellow
Early Pregnancy and Gynaecology Assessment Unit
King's College Hospital
London, UK

Wunmi Ogunnoiki, MRCOG
Consultant Obstetrician and Gynaecologist
Maidstone Hospital
Maidstone, UK

Daghni Rajasingam, MBBS, MRCOG
Locum Consultant Obstetrician and Gynaecologist
Guy's & St Thomas' Hospital
London, UK

Vijayan Valayatham, MD, MRCOG
Consultant Obstetrician and Gynaecologist
Likas Women and Child Hospital
Sabah, Malaysia

Chapter 1
Multiple Choice Questions

You should answer each statement as true [T] or false [F].

1.1 PRE-EXISTING HYPERTENSION

(a) Pre-existing hypertension always presents before 20 weeks' gestation.

(b) Endocrine causes of pre-existing hypertension include hyperaldosteronism.

(c) Women with previously uninvestigated pre-existing hypertension in pregnancy should have their serum potassium and creatinine measured.

(d) Renal disease can present with hypertension and proteinuria that is indistinguishable from pre-eclampsia.

(e) In pregnant women with pre-existing hypertension, the risk of superimposed pre-eclampsia is related to the degree of hypertension.

Answers

(a) F
(b) T
(c) T
(d) T
(e) T

Explanation

(a) Because the physiological fall in blood pressure in the first trimester can lead to a normal booking blood pressure, a high pre-pregnancy blood pressure could be masked and only present when there is a physiological rise in the third trimester.

(b) Endocrine causes of hypertension include Conn's syndrome, other causes of hyperaldosteronism (e.g. bilateral adrenal hyperplasia), Cushing's syndrome and phaeochromocytoma.

(c) This is to screen for hyperaldosteronism, which causes hypokalaemia, and pre-existing renal impairment. It is important to remember the physiological fall in serum creatinine that occurs early in gestation.

(d) Proteinuria present before 20 weeks is indicative of underlying renal disease, but if there is no record of urinalysis in early pregnancy and a women presents with hypertension and proteinuria, it could be difficult to differentiate pre-eclampsia from underlying renal disease. It should be remembered that the former is much more common and that pre-eclampsia might rarely present at very early gestations (18–24 weeks). If abnormal liver function or thrombocytopenia are present, this points towards pre-eclampsia more than renal disease.

(e) Pregnant women with severe hypertension, defined as a diastolic blood pressure >110 mmHg at <20 weeks' gestation, have a 40% risk of superimposed pre-eclampsia.

1.2 PREGNANT WOMEN WITH PRE-EXISTING HYPERTENSION

(a) Women with pre-existing hypertension are at increased risk of placental abruption.

(b) Diuretic therapy should be discontinued before conception in women with pre-existing hypertension.

(c) Proteinuria develops earlier in women with pre-existing hypertension than other women with pre-eclampsia.

(d) Antihypertensive therapy must be continued throughout pregnancy in women with pre-existing hypertension.

(e) Women with pre-existing hypertension should not breastfeed if switched back to angiotensin-converting enzyme (ACE) inhibitors after delivery.

Answers

(a) T
(b) F
(c) F
(d) F
(e) F

Explanation

(a) Women with pre-existing hypertension are at increased risk of placental abruption, even if they do not develop superimposed pre-eclampsia.

(b) There is no need to discontinue diuretics before conception; they are not thought to be teratogenic. The reason why diuretics are normally discontinued in pregnancy is because they could confound the picture in pre-eclampsia, causing volume depletion in an already vasoconstricted state. They can be safely used in pregnancy to treat pulmonary oedema, fluid overload and benign intracranial hypertension.

(c) There is no reason why women with pre-existing hypertension would develop proteinuria at earlier gestations. If they have underlying renal disease, they might already have significant proteinuria before the development of pre-eclampsia, making pre-eclampsia more difficult to diagnose.

(d) Because blood pressure usually falls in the first half of pregnancy, even in hypertensive women, this might enable the temporary withdrawal of antihypertensive therapy, especially in women who only require a low dose of one drug to control their hypertension outside pregnancy. It is usual to need to reinstitute antihypertensive therapy later in pregnancy, particularly after 28 weeks, when the physiological effect is for blood pressure to increase again.

(e) Although ACE inhibitors are contraindicated in pregnancy, they can be safely used by breastfeeding mothers.

1.3 PRE-ECLAMPSIA

(a) Pre-eclampsia can cause disseminated intravascular coagulopathy (DIC).

(b) If pre-eclampsia necessitates delivery prior to 34 weeks' gestation, screening for antiphospholipid syndrome is indicated.

(c) Pre-eclampsia commonly necessitates the use of antihypertensive agents in the puerperium.

(d) Use of low-dose aspirin does not reduce pre-eclampsia.

(e) Pre-eclampsia predisposes to pulmonary oedema.

Answers

(a) T
(b) T
(c) T
(d) F
(e) T

Explanation

(a) DIC is an unusual, but recognised, complication of pre-eclampsia. It can occur in up to 20% of cases of HELLP (haemolysis, elevated liver enzymes, low platelets) syndrome, but is more common if there is placental abruption or haemorrhage from other causes.

(b) The diagnostic criteria for antiphospholipid syndrome include one or more premature births (<34 weeks' gestation), with normal fetal morphology, due to pre-eclampsia or severe placental insufficiency.

(c) Antihypertensive agents are required postpartum in more than 60% of women with pre-eclampsia, and more commonly in those who antenatally have heavy proteinuria or severe hypertension or require antihypertensive agents or preterm delivery.

(d) Meta analyis of large randomised, controlled trials shows that low dose aspirin [75 mg daily] reduces the risk of developing pre-eclampsia by 19% [1].

(e) Women with pre-eclampsia have leaky capillaries and hypoalbuminaemia. They are, therefore, particularly vulnerable to fluid overload and pulmonary oedema, which most commonly presents postpartum but can occur antenatally.

1.4 MATERNAL SUPRAVENTRICULAR TACHYCARDIA

The following drugs would be appropriate and safe to treat a maternal supraventricular tachycardia (SVT) at 27 weeks' gestation:

(a) Verapamil
(b) Digoxin
(c) Adenosine
(d) Amiodarone
(e) Flecanide

Answers

(a) T
(b) T
(c) T
(d) F
(e) T

Explanation

The first-choice therapy for SVT is usually nonpharmacological, using vagal manoeuvres such as carotid sinus massage, eyeball pressure or sudden immersion of the face in cold water. If medical therapy is needed, adenosine is the first-line treatment, but if cardioversion does not result with intravenous adenosine, alternative options include verapamil. For prevention of further attacks, the first choice in pregnancy would be a beta-blocker such as propranolol or sotalol.

(a) Verapamil is not teratogenic. Oral use to prevent SVT in pregnancy is safe, although the intravenous formulation should be avoided or used with caution because of the risk of profound maternal hypotension. It should not normally be used in conjunction with beta-blockers. This would not, therefore, be the ideal choice for the acute management of SVT.

(b) Digoxin crosses the placenta readily but is not teratogenic. There is extensive experience of its use in pregnancy. Higher doses might be needed because of increased renal excretion in pregnancy. Digoxin reduces conductivity within the atrioventricular node. It is particularly useful to control the ventricular response in atrial fibrillation, but would not be the ideal choice for acute management of SVT.

(c) Adenosine is the treatment of choice for terminating paroxysmal SVT and usually leads to rapid reversion to sinus rhythm. Once conservative manoeuvres to induce vagal stimulation (such as carotid sinus massage and the Valsalva manoeuvre) have been tried without success, adenosine should be administered by rapid intravenous injection in increments every 1–2 minutes. The starting dose is 3 mg, followed by 6 mg and then the maximal bolus dose of 12 mg. Adenosine should be given only if cardiac monitoring facilities are available. Adenosine use in pregnancy is safe and the half-life is only 7–10 seconds. Side effects, such as chest pain and dyspnoea, are therefore short-lived.

(d) Amiodarone is used to treat SVT and ventricular tachycardia. Given intravenously, it acts rapidly and is used when other drugs are ineffective or contraindicated. Amiodarone does not cause myocardial depression, but is contraindicated in pregnancy. Amiodarone structurally resembles thyroid hormones and contains iodine. Up to 15% of patients develop amiodarone-induced hypothyroidism or hyperthyroidism. Both amiodarone and its active metabolite, desmethylamiodarone, cross the placenta. The risk of fetal or neonatal hypothyroidism and growth restriction is up to 20%. Amiodarone is highly lipid-soluble and crosses readily into breast milk. Because it has a very long half-life, breast milk could contain substantial amounts of amiodarone, even if discontinued before delivery.

(e) Flecanide is widely used for the treatment of fetal tachycardia. On the basis of limited literature, which includes case reports of first-trimester exposure, its use in pregnancy seems safe. There are far more data regarding, and is more confidence in, its use in the second and third trimesters. It is used to treat arrhythmias associated with Wolff–Parkinson–White (WPW) syndrome and similar conditions with accessory pathways. It would not be the drug of first choice to treat SVT.

1.5 PROPHYLAXIS OF ENDOCARDITIS

The following require antibiotic prophylaxis for endocarditis during delivery:

(a) Ventricular septal defect (VSD)
(b) Atrial septal defect
(c) Prosthetic mitral valve
(d) Bicuspid aortic valve
(e) WPW syndrome

Answers

(a) T
(b) F
(c) T
(d) T
(e) F

Explanation

(a) If a VSD is untreated, the risk of endocarditis is significant. Appropriate antibiotic prophylaxis during delivery is as follows: intravenous amoxicillin (amoxycillin), 2 g (or intravenous vancomycin, 1 g in patients who are allergic to penicillin) and intravenous gentamicin, 120 mg (1.5 mg/kg body weight) at the induction of anaesthesia or at the onset of labour or ruptured membranes, followed by oral amoxicillin 6 hours later.
(b) Isolated ostium secundum atrial septal defects do not constitute a risk for endocarditis.
(c) The risk of endocarditis with metal prosthetic valves is significant and antibiotic prophylaxis is mandatory.
(d) Many of these patients are not diagnosed, but a bicuspid aortic valve is a common underlying feature in fatal cases of endocarditis in pregnancy in the Report on Confidential Enquiries into Maternal Deaths [2].
(e) An accessory pathway in itself is not an indication for prophylaxis of endocarditis. In practice, some women with WPW syndrome

have associated structural congenital heart defects or the pathway might have arisen as a result of the surgical correction of congenital heart disease.

1.6 THROMBOEMBOLIC DISEASE IN PREGNANCY

(a) D-dimer measurement is more useful in the management of thromboembolic disease in pregnancy than outside pregnancy.
(b) Heparin-induced thrombocytopenia (HIT) is associated with an increased risk of thrombosis.
(c) Low-molecular-weight heparin (LMWH) is less likely to cause osteopenia than unfractionated heparin (UH).
(d) An epidural should not be sited for at least 12 hours after a dose of UH.
(e) Warfarin should not be taken during lactation.

Answers

(a) F
(b) T
(c) T
(d) F
(e) F

Explanation

(a) D-dimers are commonly increased in normal pregnancy because of the prothrombotic tendency. The diagnosis of thromboembolic disease should be made on the basis of clinical findings and imaging results.
(b) HIT is extremely rare in pregnancy if a LMWH is used. With UH, it occurs most commonly in the first 10 days of treatment. HIT is part of an allergic response in which platelets are consumed and thrombosis initiated. If HIT occurs, heparin must be discontinued and an alternative treatment sought (e.g. aspirin and stockings for women at low risk, danaparoid for women at higher risk and, possibly, warfarin for those at highest risk of thromboembolic disease).
(c) The risk of an osteoporotic fracture with a LMWH is estimated at 0.04% of all pregnancies, but is probably lower than this. UH has a 2% risk of an osteoporotic fracture.
(d) UH has a short half-life, and therefore anaesthetists are usually prepared to site an epidural 4 hours after a thromboprophylactic

dose. Most anaesthetists require a 12-hour window after a thromboprophylactic dose of a LMWH and a 24-hour window for a treatment dose of a LMWH.

(e) Warfarin is safe to use in breastfeeding women.

1.7 DEEP VEIN THROMBOSIS

(a) Deep vein thrombosis (DVT) is twice as common in pregnant women compared with women who are not pregnant.
(b) DVT is more common in the third trimester than the first.
(c) In pregnancy, DVT is more common in the right leg than the left.
(d) Venous ulceration is occasionally caused by DVT.
(e) Patients with DVT have a 1% risk of development of a pulmonary embolus.

Answers

(a) F
(b) F
(c) F
(d) F
(e) T

Explanation

(a) In pregnancy the risk of thromboembolic disease is six fold greater than the nonpregnant population.
(b) The increase in thromboembolic events starts early in the first trimester and is not related to gestational age. The risk increases again in the puerperium because of the increased likelihood of immobilization, dehydration, infection and pelvic trauma. All three arms of Virchow's triad are fulfilled, namely stasis secondary to vasodilatation and pressure from the gravid uterus, increased coagulation factors (as part of the body's adaptation to minimize haemorrhage there is an oestrogen-driven increase in clotting-factor production) and endothelial damage (especially during miscarriage, termination, surgery for ectopic pregnancy and both vaginal and Caesarean delivery).
(c) In pregnancy 85% of DVTs occur in the left leg. This is because of the anatomical arrangement of the pelvic veins, whereby the left iliac vein is compressed by the right iliac artery as it arises

from the aorta, which is itself to the left of the inferior vena cava.

(d) Following DVT, women should wear a full-length support stocking for 2 years, in order to minimize the relatively high risk of venous insufficiency and, consequently, venous ulceration. This risk is generally quoted as between 5% and 10%.

(e) Pulmonary embolus is a leading cause of maternal mortality. Although the absolute incidence is low, thromboprophylaxis and correct treatment of acute DVT are important for minimizing this risk.

1.8 TREATMENT OPTIONS FOR DIABETES IN PREGNANCY

(a) Gliclazide is teratogenic.

(b) Angiotensin converting enzyme (ACE) inhibitors should be stopped in the second trimester.

(c) Folate (5 mg/day) should be taken before conception and for the first trimester.

(d) A basal bolus regimen gives better neonatal outcome than twice-daily premixed insulin.

(e) Postprandial testing of glucose enables tighter control of diabetes than preprandial testing.

Answers

(a) F
(b) F
(c) T
(d) T
(e) T

Explanation

(a) The leading cause of teratogenesis in diabetic pregnancy is poor glycaemic control at conception. There are not extensive studies on the use of sulphonylureas in the first trimester of pregnancy. However, in clinical practice, preconception advice should be based on achieving optimal diabetic control, and if this can be done with gliclazide, then the drug does not need to be discontinued until the pregnancy test is positive. For many women, however, insulin therapy is required before conception, in order to achieve adequate control.

(b) ACE inhibitors are taken by many women with diabetic renal disease to slow the disease progression. There is increasing evidence of adverse fetal renal effects and major congenital malformation, and so ideally they should be stopped prior to conception or as soon as possible thereafter.

(c) "High-dose" folate (5 mg/day) should be taken before conception by women with established diabetes. This is a guideline from the Scottish Intercollegiate Guidelines Network (SIGN) [4] and Confidential Enquiry into Maternal and Child Health (CEMACH). In the recent CEMACH survey of pregnancy in women with established diabetes 2002–03 [5], only 40% of women achieved this. As in earlier studies, neural tube defects (NTDs) occurred about four times more often in diabetic pregnancy than expected in the general population. Other women at increased risk of NTDs, such as those taking anticonvulsant agents and those with a personal or family history of pregnancy complicated by NTDs, should also take folate at this dose.

(d) In diabetic pregnancy, neonatal outcome is influenced by structural anomaly, prematurity, growth restriction in the presence of microvascular disease or pre-eclampsia, birth trauma secondary to accelerated growth, neonatal hypoglycaemia, jaundice, polycythaemia and left-ventricular hypertrophy. All of these can be improved, or the risk reduced, by tight diabetic control. The Diabetes Control and Complication Trial (DCCT) provided useful information on the advantages of tight diabetic control in pregnancy [6]. A basal bolus (short-acting insulin with each meal and long-acting insulin overnight and/or each morning) gives better control for most women than twice-daily premixed insulins, which contain fixed ratios of short-acting and long-acting insulin.

(e) There is some evidence that measurement of blood glucose levels 2 hours postprandially gives better control than premeal tests [7]. The logic is that hyperglycaemia is the main determinant of adverse neonatal outcome in diabetic pregnancy, and, therefore, glycaemic control must include assessments when the levels are highest. By recording these postmeal values, subsequent changes to the insulin doses preceding meals can be made, with the aim of enhancing control. By definition, premeal tests record the glucose nadirs. Although it is important that these levels are also optimized, these alone are no longer accepted as sufficient monitoring, which must incorporate both premeal and postmeal measurements.

1.9 WOMEN WITH ESTABLISHED DIABETES

(a) There is an increased risk of aneuploidy in the offspring of diabetic women.

(b) The risk of structural congenital anomaly depends on glycaemic control at conception in women with established diabetes.

(c) Neonates of women with established diabetes have an increased risk of jaundice.

(d) The offspring are more likely to develop type 1 diabetes if the mother has type 1 diabetes than if the father has type 1 diabetes.

(e) The risk of pre-eclampsia is increased in women with established diabetes.

(f) Heartburn can indicate autonomic neuropathy in women with diabetes.

(g) Women with type 2 diabetes have a better pregnancy outcome than those with type 1 diabetes.

Answers

(a) F
(b) T
(c) T
(d) F
(e) T
(f) T
(g) F

Explanation

(a) Diabetes does not influence the risk of aneuploidy, which is largely determined by maternal age. However, maternal response to an aneuploid pregnancy could be affected by her diabetes – e.g. if her own quality of life or life expectancy are impaired by diabetes, she might feel it is less appropriate to have a handicapped child; her decision to terminate an aneuploid pregnancy rather than allow nature to take its inevitable course might be influenced by the difficulties of achieving good diabetic control.

(b) There are good data that the glycosylated haemoglobin (HbA_{1c}) level at conception has a strong influence on the risk of a structural anomaly in the fetus. If HbA_{1c} is normal, the risk of an anomaly is the same as in the general population, approximately 2–3%. If HbA_{1c} is over 10%, the risk of an anomaly is at least 30%, and possibly more. Because most structural anomalies occur in the first 8 weeks of the pregnancy (e.g. NTDs at 5–6 weeks and heart defects at 8 weeks), glycaemic control must be optimized before conception.

(c) Jaundice is more common in babies of diabetic women. It is proposed that fetal hyperinsulinaemia results in increased fetal erythropoietin production, which in turn causes neonatal poly-cythaemia. Breakdown of some of these excess red blood cells and immature liver enzymes, for handling the bilirubin load, pre-dispose these babies to jaundice. It is estimated that about 20% develop jaundice.

(d) In type 1 diabetes, the fetus has a higher chance of developing dia-betes if the father is affected, rather than if the mother is affected. The cumulative risk of developing diabetes by the age of 20 years for children with mothers who have type 1 diabetes is 1.4–5%, approximately 10–30 times greater than background. The risk is only one-third of that if the father (rather than the mother) has the disease. This is postulated to be because of in-utero development of tolerance to pancreatic beta-cell autoantigens if the mother has diabetes; it is not because of the demise of susceptible fetuses. Interestingly, children whose mothers have type 1 diabetes could have an increased risk of type 2 diabetes, which is ascribed to fuel-mediated intrauterine events causing fetal hyperinsulinism [8].

(e) Women with established diabetes do have an increased inci-dence of pre-eclampsia, and this is raised further if they have pre-existing hypertension or diabetic renal disease.

(f) Autonomic neuropathy is not a common problem in diabetic pregnancy. However, it can cause postural hypotension and delayed gastric emptying with severe nausea, vomiting and reflux oesophagitis.

(g) In the CEMACH report [5], the perinatal mortality was as high for women with type 2 as those with type 1 diabetes.

1.10 GESTATIONAL DIABETES

(a) Women have a 50% risk of developing type 2 diabetes later in life.
(b) Women have a 75% chance of developing gestational diabetes in a subsequent pregnancy.
(c) Weight loss and exercise reduce insulin resistance.
(d) Shoulder dystocia can be predicted by antenatal ultrasound measurements.
(e) Insulin should be continued until the baby is at least 12 hours of age.

Answers

(a) T
(b) F
(c) T

(d) F
(e) F

Explanation

(a) Gestational diabetes can be considered a "stress test" of insulin metabolism. In normal pregnancy, insulin production doubles and peripheral insulin resistance develops, with the dual processes of "accelerated starvation" and "facilitated anabolism". Women who cannot make these metabolic changes are inherently more likely to develop diabetes in later life. Being pregnant does not in itself alter the risk of subsequent diabetes.

(b) In subsequent pregnancies the chance of gestational diabetes developing again is over 90%, unless there has been substantial weight loss.

(c) Women should have lifelong intentions to attain an ideal body weight and exercise regularly, because both reduce insulin resistance and so improve glucose metabolism.

(d) Shoulder dystocia is difficult to predict. Serial antenatal ultrasound measurements showing accelerated growth indicate an increased risk but has a low positive-predictive value, and the absence of this picture has a poor negative-predictive value. It is reasonable obstetric practice to have an experienced obstetrician available for the delivery of all babies whose mothers have required insulin during pregnancy.

(e) Insulin requirements return to prepregnancy levels as soon as delivery is complete. Insulin treatment should be discontinued straight away, in order to avoid hypoglycaemia. If labour has been rapid and delivery completed within the duration of action of antenatally administered long-acting insulin, special care should be taken to avoid hypoglycaemia.

1.11 POSTNATAL CARE OF WOMEN WITH DIABETES

Ms A is 29 years old. She has had type 1 diabetes mellitus since she was 6 years old, which is generally well controlled, with no evidence of end-organ damage; she is otherwise fit and well, and is a slim nonsmoker. She has just delivered her first child after an intensely managed, but largely uncomplicated, pregnancy and labour; she does not want to conceive again for "ages". You review her on the postnatal ward on the morning after her spontaneous vaginal delivery:

(a) She can take enalapril, even if she continues with breastfeeding.

(b) She can use the combined oral contraceptive pill (COCP) once breastfeeding is complete.

(c) Her total insulin dose during lactation is likely to be higher than her normal nonpregnant dose.

(d) Depot Provera is relatively contraindicated because of the diabetes.

(e) She does not require postnatal thromboprophylaxis.

Answers

(a) T
(b) F
(c) F
(d) T
(e) T

Explanation

(a) Enalapril is an ACE inhibitor used in patients with diabetes to slow deterioration of renal function. It seems to be safe in lactation and can be started soon after delivery, as required. The drug should not be prescribed during pregnancy because it affects the fetal renal tract, causing impaired nephron migration in the first trimester and fetal renal artery vasoconstriction in the second half of pregnancy, with consequent oligohydramnios and its associated complications. It is also teratogenic [3].

(b) The World Health Organization (WHO) lists the use of the COCP in women with diabetes of 20-years' duration or more as category 3/4 – i.e. either the risks outweigh the advantages of use (category 3) or the use is absolutely contraindicated (category 4). The combined hormonal contraceptive patches (e.g. Evra) fall under the same classification as the COCP.

(c) Insulin regimens are normally approximately 25% less during breastfeeding compared with the usual nonpregnant dose. Lactation requires around 1000–1500 kcal/day. In addition, breastfeeding women are more active at night than when they are not breastfeeding and therefore must avoid hypoglycaemia.

(d) The WHO lists use of depot Provera as category 3. The concerns relate to the increased risk of cardiovascular complications. The potential for unpredictable return of fertility following use of depot Provera is a further disadvantage: women with diabetes should achieve optimal diabetic control before conception, and need a form of contraception that enables their fertility to return to normal quickly when it is discontinued. Contraception is important for this lady, and should be reliable. She could consider the progesterone only pill (POP) if she can manage the strict regimen (although using Cerazette obviates this because it has a 12-hour window, rather than the 3-hour window of other POPs) or a progestogen implant (e.g. Implanon), progestogen-releasing intrauterine system (e.g. Mirena) or copper intrauterine contraceptive device. The low and steady dose of progestogen from these two hormonal options does not increase the risk of cardiovascular complications [9].

(e) Thromboprophylaxis should be considered for women with diabetes during pregnancy and the puerperium. This patient does not seem to have any additional risk factors for thrombosis (she is slim, young and a nonsmoker), and she had an uncomplicated vaginal delivery. Therefore, she does not need postnatal thromboprophylaxis.

1.12 THROMBOCYTOPENIA

The following can cause a maternal platelet count less than 100×10^9 platelets/l in pregnancy:

(a) Human immunodeficiency virus (HIV)
(b) Thrombosis
(c) Haemorrhage
(d) Endometritis
(e) Alloimmune thrombocytopenia

Answers

(a) T
(b) F
(c) T
(d) T
(e) F

Explanation

(a) HIV can present with anaemia, leucopenia, thrombocytopenia or pancytopenia. A low platelet count at booking should always prompt consideration of HIV.
(b) A low platelet count is not a feature of acute thrombosis. A high platelet count could cause thrombosis.
(c) Haemorrhage could lead to thrombocytopenia either because of the development of DIC and consumption of clotting factors or after blood transfusion.

(d) Any cause of sepsis, either antenatal or postnatal, could be associated with thrombocytopenia.
(e) Alloimmune thrombocytopenia is a cause of fetal, not maternal, thrombocytopenia. The maternal platelet count is normal in this condition.

Other causes of thrombocytopenia in pregnancy include gestational thrombocytopenia, pre-eclampsia, antiphospholipid syndrome, immune thrombocytopenic purpura (ITP), thrombotic thrombocytopenic purpura (TTP) and haemolytic uraemic syndrome (HUS).

1.13 FOLATE SUPPLEMENTATION

The following conditions are indications for treatment with folic acid (5 mg/day) in pregnancy:

(a) Hereditary spherocytosis
(b) Sulfasalazine therapy
(c) Carbamezepine therapy
(d) Vegetarian diet
(e) Sickle cell disease

Answers

(a) T
(b) T
(c) T
(d) F
(e) T

Explanation

(a) Any haemolytic anaemia could lead to folate deficiency. Both sickle cell disease and hereditary spherocytosis are haemolytic anaemias.
(b) Sulfasalazine has antifolate actions and is a dihydrofolate reductase inhibitor. It is, therefore, associated with an increased risk of NTDs, oral clefts and cardiovascular defects. Folate (5 mg/day) supplementation is recommended throughout pregnancy.
(c) Carbamezepine is an antiepileptic drug that is associated with an increased risk of congenital malformations, particularly NTDs, and folate-deficiency anaemia.
(d) Vegetarians are not usually folate-deficient as fruit and vegetables are folate-rich unless they have been over cooked.
(e) See part (a).

1.14 NEUROPATHIES AND PALSIES IN PREGNANCY

The following nerves might be affected by neuropathies or palsies in pregnancy:

(a) Lateral cutaneous nerve of the thigh
(b) Optic nerve
(c) Facial nerve
(d) Hypoglossal nerve
(e) Median nerve

Answers

(a) T
(b) F
(c) T
(d) F
(e) T

Explanation

(a) The lateral cutaneous nerve of the thigh, supplying sensation to the outer aspect of the thigh, might be compressed by the gravid abdomen as the nerve passes behind or through the inguinal ligament, medial to the anterior superior iliac spine.
(b) The optic nerve is not affected by neuropathies or palsies in pregnancy.
(c) Bell's palsy, caused by a lower motor neurone lesion of the facial (VIIth cranial) nerve, is more common in pregnant women than nonpregnant women. Oedema around the nerve causes compression as it exits the skull through the stylomastoid foramen, sometimes in association with herpes virus infection.
(d) The hypoglossal nerve, or XIIth cranial nerve, supplies the muscles of the tongue and is no more commonly affected in pregnancy than outside pregnancy.
(e) Compression of the median nerve as it passes through the carpal tunnel is well recognised as a common complication of pregnancy, possibly related to oedema.

1.15 EPILEPSY

(a) Free drug levels of carbamezepine fall during pregnancy.
(b) The recommended preconceptual dose of folic acid for women taking anticonvulsants is the same as that for women with a previous child with a NTD.

(c) Women taking sodium valproate should be advised not to breastfeed.
(d) Vigabatrin is not teratogenic.
(e) The risk of epileptic seizures increases intrapartum.

Answers

(a) T
(b) T
(c) F
(d) F
(e) T

Explanation

(a) Because of the increased blood volume and resulting increased volume of distribution, in addition to increased excretion of drugs through the liver and kidney, free drug levels of most antiepileptic drugs fall in pregnancy. For many women carbamezepine does not have a narrow therapeutic window and so dose changes are not necessarily needed. Conversely, increases in lamotrigine dose are frequently required.
(b) Women taking antiepileptic drugs before conception and in early pregnancy are advised to take folic acid (5 mg/day) to reduce the risk of NTDs and other abnormalities, such as cardiovascular and urogenital malformations.
(c) Negligible amounts of sodium valproate are found in breast milk. Only 1–10% of valproate is transferred from plasma to breast milk, and the maximum amount received by the baby is likely to be 3% of a therapeutic dose. Breastfeeding should, therefore, be encouraged.
(d) Vigabatrin is teratogenic in animals and humans, and it should be avoided if possible in pregnancy.
(e) Women with epilepsy are more likely to have seizures around the time of delivery. This is related to several factors, including hyperventilation, lack of absorption of drugs from the gastrointestinal tract during labour (which can be minimised by administering drugs intravenously or rectally), stress and lack of sleep at the end of pregnancy. The risk of seizures is about 1–2% during labour and 1–2% in the first 24 hours postpartum.

1.16 CEREBRAL VEIN THROMBOSIS

(a) Cerebral vein thrombosis might present with convulsions.
(b) Usually, cerebral vein thrombosis occurs in the third trimester.

(c) Fever and leucocytosis can be caused by cerebral vein thrombosis.
(d) In the UK, cerebral vein thrombosis is the commonest thrombotic cause of maternal death in the puerperium.
(e) If headache is associated with hemiparesis, cerebral vein thrombosis should be considered.

Answers

(a) T
(b) F
(c) T
(d) F
(e) T

Explanation

Cerebral vein thrombosis is uncommon (incidence, approximately 1 in 10,000 pregnancies per year), but associated with a high mortality. Most fatal cases (about 1 fatal case/year in the UK) related to pregnancy occur in the puerperium. Patients usually present with headache, which might be associated with seizures, impaired consciousness and signs of raised intracranial pressure, with vomiting and photophobia fever and leucocytosis are not uncommon, and the differential diagnosis for cerebral vein thrombosis therefore often includes meningitis and encephalitis. One-third to two-thirds of patients have focal signs, such as hemiparesis. Venous infarction and intracerebral bleeding can result from obstruction of the collateral circulation. Differential diagnoses include eclampsia, subarachnoid haemorrhage and herpes encephalitis. Diagnosis is made by computerised tomography scanning (CT) to detect intracerebral bleeding, although magnetic resonance imaging (MRI), especially venous angiography MRI, best shows venous clots. Treatment with heparin is controversial because the risk of intracerebral bleeding might be increased, but clot formation is prevented. Evidence suggests outcome is better with heparin therapy.

1.17 ECLAMPSIA

(a) Eclampsia is always preceded by hyperreflexia or drowsiness.
(b) The (maternal) outcome in eclampsia is related to gestation.
(c) Magnesium sulphate ($MgSO_4$) might cause respiratory arrest.
(d) In the UK, most patients with eclampsia have their first fit at home.
(e) Maternal mortality from eclampsia in the UK is 10%.

Answers

(a) F
(b) T
(c) T
(d) F
(e) F

Explanation

(a) Eclampsia might not be preceded by any classical features of pre-eclampsia, and there is no relationship between the presence of hyperreflexia and clonus and the development of eclampsia. There could be preceding headache or neurological symptoms or signs, but not necessarily.
(b) Both antepartum and preterm eclampsia are independent risk factors for a severe maternal outcome.
(c) $MgSO_4$ is the drug of choice for primary and secondary prophylaxis of eclampsia, but high serum concentrations can result in loss of tendon reflexes (>5 mmol/l) and neuromuscular paralysis (>7.5 mmol/l).
(d) The British Eclampsia Survey [10] showed 75% of patients have their first fit in hospital.
(e) Maternal mortality from eclampsia is approximately 2%.

1.18 THYROID DYSFUNCTION

When considering the treatment of thyroid dysfunction in pregnancy, the following medications should be avoided:

(a) Thyroxine in the first trimester.
(b) Propranolol in the first trimester.
(c) Radioactive iodine for 4 months before conception.
(d) Carbimazole at all gestations.
(e) Propylthiouracil (PTU) at term.

Answers

(a) F
(b) F
(c) T
(d) F
(e) F

Explanation

(a) Thyroxine is not only safe in the first trimester, but it is also important for fetal neurological development. Children whose mothers had untreated or undertreated hypothyroidism in the first trimester have a greater risk of neurodevelopmental delay than those whose mothers were correctly treated with thyroxine or were euthyroid. Beyond the first trimester, placental changes prevent significant thyroxine from crossing unless the fetus is athyrotic [11].

(b) Propranolol use is safe in the first trimester. Although atenolol might cause growth restriction if given in the first trimester, this has not been shown with propranolol and, in any case, it would not be a reason to withhold beta-blockers from a thyrotoxic patient.

(c) Iodine crosses the placenta, and radioactive iodine destroys developing thyroid tissue. The Royal College of Physicians' (RCP) guidelines recommend that it is avoided in the 4 months before conception and during pregnancy and lactation. People who are given radioactive iodine should avoid nonessential close personal contact with pregnant women and babies for up to 27 days, depending on the dose administered [12].

(d) Carbimazole and PTU can both be used with confidence throughout pregnancy when clinically indicated. They are not teratogenic, and any link with the very rare aplasia cutis is either extremely weak or co-incidental. There is also evidence that they each reduce the risk of teratogenesis that untreated, or under-treated, thyrotoxicosis brings with it [13]. Contrary to earlier dogma, sophisticated experiments on isolated term placental lobules show that carbimazole does not cross the placenta more readily than PTU. Both drugs carry a small risk of fetal hypothyroidism, so should be given at the lowest dose to maintain a clinically euthyroid state with the free thyroxine concentration (fT_4) at the upper end of normal for pregnancy.

(e) See (d).

1.19 POSTPARTUM THYROIDITIS

(a) Postpartum throiditis usually presents within 6 weeks of delivery.

(b) Symptoms of hyperthyroidism are common in postpartum thyroiditis.

(c) Hyperthyroidism can be treated with PTU.

(d) Hypothyroidism usually resolves by 6 months postpartum.

(e) There is a high risk of recurrence in future pregnancies.

Answers

(a) F
(b) F
(c) F
(d) F
(e) T

Explanation

(a) Postpartum thyroiditis is a subacute destructive autoimmune condition that is strongly related to antiperoxidase antibodies and occurs in the first year postpartum. It can present as hyperthyroidism, hypothyroidism or, most often, a purely biochemical phenomenon; the prevalence in clinical practice is much lower than the 2–17% described in clinical trials.

In clinically apparent cases, any or all of the three phases can occur: hyperthyroidism at 1–3 months postpartum, hypothyroidism at 3–8 months postpartum, and euthyroidism by 1 year postpartum.

(b) Hyperthyroidism is usually asymptomatic.

(c) If treatment is required, it is treatment of the symptoms themselves – e.g. beta-blockers for tachycardia and tremor. Thionamides are not needed because the thyrotoxic picture is due to increased release of preformed thyroxine from the damaged thyroid, rather than excess formation of thyroxine.

(d) The hypothyroid phase is more likely to be symptomatic than the hyperthyroid phase, requiring treatment, although the symptoms might be vague and difficult to distinguish from other postnatal problems. Treatment is with thyroxine. In most cases, the autoimmune process has subsided by 12 months postpartum and the thyroid gland has returned to normal: thyroxine should be withdrawn when the baby is 1 year old.

(e) Follow-up thyroid tests are important because a small proportion of women have permanent hypothyroidism and 5% of women each year subsequently develop it; 70% of women get postpartum thyroiditis following subsequent pregnancies [14,15].

1.20 PITUITARY HORMONES

The following can be said of pituitary hormones in pregnancy:

(a) The placenta secretes adrenocorticotropic hormone (ACTH).
(b) Levels of basal growth hormone (GH) are unchanged.

(c) Prolactin secretion is reduced until the onset of suckling.
(d) Follicle stimulating hormone (FSH) and luteinizing hormone (LH) levels are increased.
(e) The placenta secretes antidiuretic hormone (ADH).

Answers

(a) T
(b) T
(c) F
(d) F
(e) F

Explanation

(a) The placenta does secrete ACTH, although pituitary secretion is unchanged.
(b) Levels of basal growth hormone secretion from the pituitary are unchanged, although the placenta secretes placental GH and human placental lactogen, which is closely related to GH.
(c) Pituitary secretion of prolactin is increased throughout pregnancy so that levels 10-fold greater than those of nonpregnancy are encountered. Levels fall rapidly postpartum, unless breastfeeding commences.
(d) FSH and LH secretion are suppressed by the high levels of oestrogen in pregnancy and levels are usually undetectable.
(e) The placenta secretes vasopressinase, which metabolises ADH, occasionally producing diabetes insipidus because of ADH deficiency in late pregnancy.

1.21 PROLACTINOMAS IN PREGNANCY

(a) Microprolactinomas should be managed by continuation of dopamine agonists.
(b) Enlargement of the tumour might present with headache.
(c) Macroprolactinomas are an indication for regular visual-field testing.
(d) Cabergoline is contraindicated in pregnancy.
(e) Women with prolactinomas should be advised against breastfeeding.

Answers

(a) F
(b) T

(c) T
(d) F
(e) F

Explanation

(a) Women with microprolactinomas can usually discontinue dopamine agonists in pregnancy as the risk of expansion of the tumour is very small.
(b) Other symptoms might include visual-field defects.
(c) Macroprolactinomas are more likely to expand during pregnancy than microprolactinomas. Visual field testing is performed to detect any tumour expansion upwards, causing compression of the optic nerve or chiasm.
(d) Both bromocriptine and cabergoline can be safely taken in pregnancy and are usually electively continued in women with macroprolactinomas.
(e) There is no reason why women with prolactinomas should not breastfeed, although lactation might be suppressed in those taking dopamine agonists.

1.22 ERYTHEMA NODOSUM

Erythema nodosum is associated with the following:
(a) Streptococcal sore throat
(b) SLE
(c) Normal pregnancy
(d) Histoplasmosis
(e) Chlamydial infection

Answers

(a) T
(b) F
(c) T
(d) T
(e) T

Explanation

Erythema nodosum is a painful or tender nodule over the shin that is dusky red, purple or blue and fades over several weeks. It is most common in young women and can be idiopathic. It is also associated with tuberculosis, sarcoidosis, inflammatory bowel disease and drugs (including OCP, NSAIDs and sulphonamides).

1.23 RHEUMATOID ARTHRITIS

(a) The pregnancy outcome is related to disease activity.
(b) ESR is a useful marker of disease activity in pregnancy.
(c) New-onset weakness in the legs requires urgent assessment.
(d) Methotrexate should be stopped as soon as the pregnancy test is positive.
(e) Sulfasalazine reduces the speed of disease progression and is safe in pregnancy.

Answers

(a) F
(b) F
(c) T
(d) F
(e) T

Explanation

(a) Women with rheumatoid arthritis might experience some improvement in their symptoms during pregnancy, although up to one-quarter will continue to have severe symptoms. Unlike other autoimmune conditions, there is no evidence that disease activity influences pregnancy outcome, which is generally good unless there is hypertension, secondary antiphospholipid syndrome (APS) (uncommon), or significant joint problems that limit hip abduction (for vaginal delivery) or neck extension (for general anaesthetic).

(b) Outside pregnancy, disease activity can be monitored by elevation of ESR. However, normal pregnancy is associated with a modest elevation of ESR too, readings of 50 to 100 mm/hour being normal depending on the gestational age and haemoglobin concentration [16]. CRP should be used instead, because it is not influenced by pregnancy and, unlike SLE, disease activity does affect it.

(c) An anaesthetic opinion should be sought routinely during pregnancy for all women with rheumatoid arthritis, because upper cervical spine involvement makes intubation for general anaesthetic hazardous. Cervical spinal cord compression is rare, but constitutes a neurosurgical emergency. It might present as increased difficulty walking unrelated to joint disease, leg weakness, or loss of bowel or bladder control.

(d) Drug therapy is often one of the greatest challenges in pregnant women with rheumatoid arthritis. Analgesia should ideally be given with paracetamol-based drugs; if these are inadequate, NSAIDS can be considered in the first half of the pregnancy, but not thereafter because of the risks of fetal renal artery vasoconstriction and premature closure of the ductus arteriosus. Disease-modifying antirheumatic drugs (DMARDS) slow disease progression, but are often used in conjunction with symptomatic treatment because alone they frequently only achieve partial improvement and this is not immediate. Methotrexate, sulfasalazine, leflunamide and ciclosporin have all been shown to slow the rate of progressive joint damage. However, methotrexate is a folate antagonist that should be stopped at least 3–6 months before conception. Conception while taking methotrexate is associated with an increased risk of NTDs and other skeletal abnormalities.

(e) Sulfasalazine is safe in pregnancy, but high-dose folate (5 mg daily) must also be prescribed because the drug has an antifolate action.

1.24 INFLAMMATORY BOWEL DISEASE

The following might be seen as complications of inflammatory bowel disease in pregnancy:

(a) Ascending cholangitis
(b) Erythema nodosum
(c) Premature labour
(d) Erythema multiforme
(e) Iron-deficiency anaemia

Answers

(a) T
(b) T
(c) T
(d) T
(e) T

Explanation

(a) Ascending cholangitis is a recognised complication/association of both Crohn's disease and ulcerative colitis.

(b) Erythema nodosum might be seen in association with inflammatory bowel disease.

(c) Active inflammatory bowel disease is associated with spontaneous preterm labour.

(d) Skin manifestations of inflammatory bowel disease include erythema nodosum, erythema multiforme and pyoderma gangrenosum. Erythema multiforme is an acute mucocutaneous hypersensitivity reaction, and its most common form is associated with symmetrical target lesions on the extremities.

(e) Inflammatory bowel disease might cause a normochromic normocytic anaemia of chronic disorder, a microcytic anaemia of iron deficiency secondary to blood loss or a macrocytic picture because of malabsorption of vitamin B12 from the terminal ileum.

1.25 ULCERATIVE COLITIS

Consider the following for a woman with ulcerative colitis who is pregnant:

(a) She should aim to stop aminosalicyclates, if possible.

(b) She has previously had a pancolectomy and, following formation of an ileal pouch, is fully continent; she should aim for a vaginal delivery if obstetric conditions permit.

(c) If she is taking steroids, check her parvovirus immune status.

(d) Backache should be investigated thoroughly.

(e) Her offspring do not have an increased risk of developing the condition.

Answers

(a) F
(b) T
(c) F
(d) T
(e) F

Explanation

(a) Maintenance of remission is important in ulcerative colitis: flares are most common in the first trimester or if treatment is inappropriately reduced or stopped. Aminosalicyclates, such as mesalazine, can be administered as foam enemas, suppositories or tablets. They are safe in pregnancy, and should only be stopped if it is certain that the disease is fully quiescent. Folate (5 mg daily) should be taken with aminosalicyclates, because they have an antifolate action.

(b) Caesarean section (LSCS) is usually best avoided in women with inflammatory bowel disease, especially if they have had bowel surgery, because the operation can be technically difficult, with an increased risk of trauma to local structures, including the bowel and bladder. In addition, women with active inflammatory bowel disease have an increased risk of thrombosis, and therefore their peripartum risk of a thromboembolic event should be minimized. Typical nonobstetric indications for LSCS might include active perianal disease if there is a risk of fistula formation, severe perineal scarring with reduced elasticity and faecal incontinence. Ileal pouches per se are not usually an indication for LSCS. However, it is clearly important that obstetric factors that could impair function of the pouch (e.g. prolonged second stage of labour and third-degree tear) and provoke incontinence are avoided.

(c) Prednisolone administration in pregnancy is generally safer than a severe relapse, and should be used to treat flares of ulcerative colitis. Maternal side effects of steroid courses lasting longer than 2–3 weeks include hypertension, hyperglycaemia and Addisonian collapse if additional doses are not prescribed during stressful episodes (such as labour). In addition, if chickenpox develops, there is an increased incidence of the serious complications of this infection, including pneumonitis and encephalitis: women should have their immune status checked. There is not an increased risk of parvovirus infection.

(d) Backache in pregnancy has a broad differential diagnosis, and is often benign. In a woman with ulcerative colitis consider ankylosing spondylitis and vertebral collapse because of steroid-induced osteoporosis.

(e) Clustering of cases occurs, and is more common in certain ethnic groups.

1.26 HYPEREMESIS GRAVIDARUM

The following intravenous fluids are appropriate in the management of hyperemesis gravidarum:

(a) Hartmann's solution
(b) Double-strength normal saline
(c) 5% dextrose solution
(d) 10% dextrose solution
(e) Normal saline

Answers

(a) T
(b) F

(c) F
(d) F
(e) T

Explanation

Women with prolonged recurrent vomiting are usually hypona-traemic and volume-depleted. They are prone to both Wernicke's encephalopathy, because of thiamine deficiency, and central pontine myelinolysis, because of severe hyponatraemia or its overzealous correction. Therefore, hyponatraemia should be corrected slowly with normal saline rather than double-strength saline, or Hartmanns' solution which contains physiological amounts of sodium. Dextrose (either 5% or 10%) solution contains no sodium ions and therefore exacerbates any hyponatraemia. Furthermore, solutions containing a high concentration of dextrose can precipitate Wernicke's encephalopathy if administered before thiamine replacement.

1.27 THE LIVER IN PREGNANCY

(a) Blood flow to the liver increases.
(b) Placental alkaline phosphatase is heat stable.
(c) A palpable liver edge is usually pathological.
(d) Spider naevi do not suggest chronic liver disease.
(e) Increased production of albumin occurs.

Answers

(a) F
(b) T
(c) T
(d) T
(e) F

Explanation

(a) In pregnancy, the circulating volume increases by about 50%, with a large part of this increase going to the uteroplacental circulation, kidneys and breasts. The absolute amount of blood going to the liver remains unchanged. As a percentage of cardiac output, it falls from 35% to 29% by late pregnancy.

(b) Alkaline phosphatase is produced by the liver, the placenta and bone. In pregnancy, placental production increases, especially in the third trimester, so that by term, total levels might be three times the upper limit of normal. Liver and placental isoenzymes can be distinguished by heat treatment to 60°C for 10 minutes, which destroys the liver isoenzyme (and, in adults, small amount of bone isoenzyme): in clinical practice, the amount by which the alkaline phosphatase assay falls after heat treatment can usually be considered to be the liver component.

(c) The size of the liver is unchanged in pregnancy, but it usually occupies a more superior and posterior position, such that if it is palpable, there is usually significant pathology.

(d) The characteristic lesions of chronic liver disease include spider naevi, palmar erythema and peripheral oedema, but each of these is common in normal pregnancy, the first two signs reflecting raised circulating oestrogen levels.

(e) Although liver production of some proteins increases in pregnancy, such as coagulation factors and hormone-binding proteins, albumin production is unchanged. Circulating albumin concentrations fall in normal pregnancy because of haemodilution.

1.28 ACUTE FATTY LIVER OF PREGNANCY (AFLP)

(a) AFLP usually presents near term.
(b) There is a 25% recurrence risk in some families.
(c) Itching is a feature of AFLP.
(d) Hypoglycaemia can occur.
(e) Hyperuricaemia is a feature of AFLP.

Answers

(a) T
(b) T
(c) T
(d) T
(e) T

Explanation

(a) AFLP typically presents in the third trimester.
(b) Some cases of AFLP are caused by long-chain hydroxyacyl co-enzyme A dehydrogenase (LCHAD) deficiency, a homozygous

long-chain fatty-acid metabolic problem occurring in the fetus. The fetal abnormal fatty-acid metabolites cross into the maternal circulation and overwhelm the maternal heterozygote capacity, resulting in the clinical scenario of AFLP. In these families, there is a 25% recurrence risk as for other autosomal recessive conditions, although the severity is variable. In most women, the aetiology is unclear and the risk of recurrence is low.

(c) Pruritus is a nonspecific feature of many types of liver disease, including AFLP. It is important that obstetricians do not immediately assume that itching in pregnancy is because of obstetric cholestasis.

(d) Liver failure results in impaired mobilization of glucose from the liver during fasting. In AFLP, regular blood glucose measurements should be made, and low results treated with intravenous high-concentration glucose.

(e) Hyperuricaemia is a feature of severe liver disease; in AFLP, the raised uric acid level is out of proportion with the features of pre-eclampsia, which are usually mild.

1.29 HEPATITIS C INFECTION

(a) 80% of infected individuals become chronic carriers of hepatitis C.
(b) 10% of hepatitis C carriers develop hepatoma.
(c) Materno-fetal transfer of hepatitis C infection is more likely if the mother is also HIV positive.
(d) Caesarean section should be offered to reduce the risk of fetal infection.
(e) Lactation is best avoided in women with hepatitis C infection.
(f) Sexual transmission of hepatitis C is common.

Answers

(a) T
(b) F
(c) T
(d) F
(e) F
(f) F

Explanation

(a) Hepatitis C is an RNA virus transmitted by blood and blood products, which is therefore common among intravenous drug abusers. At least 80% of infected people become carriers and develop chronic liver disease.

(b) Cirrhosis develops in approximately 20% of hepatitis C carriers over 10 years, and of these, around 10% develop primary hepatocellular carcinoma.

(c) Overall, materno-fetal vertical transmission is rare, but it seems to depend on the viraemic load. Transmission in HIV-positive women is higher, and this might reflect the propensity for higher viraemic loads.

(d) In HIV-negative hepatitis-C-positive women, there is no benefit in offering Caesarean section. However, if the viraemic load is very high, delivery by Caesarean section has been suggested to protect the neonate from infection: this area needs further study.

(e) In HIV-negative women, breastfeeding should be encouraged. Horizontal transmission of hepatitis C within the family seems to be rare.

(f) Hepatitis C is common among those with haemophilia and intravenous drug abusers. It is, however, not common in prostitutes, homosexual men and those attending sexual-health clinics, making sexual transmission unlikely.

1.30 SCLEROSING CHOLANGITIS IN PREGNANCY

(a) 25% of patients with sclerosing cholangitis in pregnancy have inflammatory bowel disease.

(b) Sclerosing cholangitis should be part of the differential diagnosis for obstetric cholestasis.

(c) Raised alkaline phosphatase supports the diagnosis of sclerosing cholangitis.

(d) Antimitochondrial antibodies might be positive in patients with sclerosing cholangitis in pregnancy.

(e) Ursodeoxycholic acid (UDCA) is a potential treatment for sclerosing cholangitis.

Answers

(a) F
(b) T
(c) F
(d) F
(e) T

Explanation

(a) Primary sclerosing cholangitis is a chronic liver disease characterized by fibrosis and inflammation in the intrahepatic and extrahepatic bile ducts. Of patients with sclerosing cholangitis, 75% have inflammatory bowel disease, usually ulcerative colitis; screening of asymptomatic patients with inflammatory bowel disease can detect an early phase of abnormal liver biochemistry.

(b) Symptoms include fluctuating pruritus (and hence the differential diagnosis in pregnancy includes obstetric cholestasis), jaundice, fever and biliary colic.

(c) Typically, liver function tests show a raised alkaline phosphatase level. However, in pregnancy, alkaline phosphatase might be three times the upper limit of normal, and therefore in this circumstance this is not such a helpful test, unless heat treatment or isoenzyme assay are available.

(d) The diagnosis is made in the presence of antinuclear cytoplasmic antibodies antimitochondrial antibodies suggest primary biliary cirrhosis, and typical cholangiogram and biopsy features.

(e) UDCA causes some transient improvement in liver function, but does not seem to alter long-term prognosis. Ultimately, liver transplantation is required.

1.31 TUBERCULOSIS IN PREGNANCY IN UK

(a) TB in pregnancy is more common in Asian and African immigrants than in indigenous women.

(b) Extrapulmonary TB is rare compared with pulmonary TB.

(c) Heaf testing is contraindicated in pregnancy.

(d) Antituberculous medication, including rifampicin, should not be used in the first trimester of pregnancy.

(e) Most cases of tuberculosis (TB) in pregnancy are associated with HIV infection.

Answers

(a) T
(b) F
(c) F
(d) F
(e) F

Explanation

(a) The prevalence of TB in UK is rising. In most UK populations, TB is typically found in recently arrived immigrants from the Asian subcontinent or Africa.

(b) Symptoms are often atypical or reported late, and the diagnosis can be challenging. Nonspecific abdominal or back pain, lymphadenopathy and respiratory symptoms should be considered seriously, especially in high-risk women. Extrapulmonary TB is common in pregnancy, accounting for more than 50% cases in two recent UK series [17].

(c) Chest X-ray helps to diagnose pulmonary TB and, with fetal shielding is safe. Serial sputa or early morning urine samples lead to a microbiological diagnosis and correct sensitivities. A Heaf test, consisting of a six-point, disposable puncture apparatus that is activated through a small amount of purified protein derivative of *Mycobacterium tuberculosis* (PPD), placed on the flexor surface of the left forearm can be used safely in pregnancy: a negative result of discrete induration at the puncture sites is classified as grade 0 or 1 (maximum, grade 4) and implies that further investigation is not required. HIV-positive patients might have a delayed response, and false negatives are more common in this population.

(d) Antituberculous medication should be used at whatever gestation of pregnancy the diagnosis of TB is made. Common regimens include rifampicin, isoniazid, ethambutol and pyrazinamide, all of which are safe throughout pregnancy and lactation.

(e) In UK, most pregnant women with TB are HIV negative.

1.32 RADIATION

(a) Almost all man-made radiation results from diagnostic medical exposures.

(b) A single PA chest X-ray is equivalent to approximately 3 days of natural background radiation.

(c) A pelvic CT scan performed in pregnancy doubles the risk of fatal childhood cancer.

(d) The threshold for gross fetal malformation caused by X-ray exposure in the first trimester is equivalent to 20 abdominal X-rays.

(e) The risk of heritable effects because of fetal irradiation (i.e. effects that could be passed on to the descendants of the unborn child) is similar to the increased risk of childhood cancers that irradiation causes.

Answers

(a) T
(b) T
(c) T
(d) F
(e) T

Explanation

(a) Man-made radiation accounts for 15% of the total radiation burden, of which 97% results from diagnostic medical procedures [18 RCR London 1995].

(b) A chest X-ray gives an effective dose of 0.002 mSv and a fetal dose of <0.001 mGy. The units of radiation can be confusing: Grays (Gy) are the absorbed dose of ionizing radiation, where 1 Gy = 1 J of energy being imparted to 1 kg of matter (previously called a Rad), and Sieverts (Sv) are a dose-equivalent of 1 J/kg (previously called the rem), where the dose-equivalent is the measure of effects of radiation on living organisms. Sieverts are calculated as the absorbed dose in Gy multiplied by the relative biological effectiveness – e.g. alpha radiation causes 20 times more biological damage than beta radiation. Humans can absorb up to 0.25 Sv without any immediate effect; 1 Sv causes radiation sickness and >8 Sv is fatal.

(c) The baseline risk of childhood cancer in the first 15 years of life is 1 in 650, and half of these cases (1 in 1300) are fatal. It is estimated that fetal exposure to X-rays increases the risk of fatal cancer in childhood by 1 in 33,000 per 1 mGy exposure. A pelvic CT scan gives an approximate fetal radiation dose of 25 mGy, which increases the risk of fatal childhood cancer to 1 in 1320. By contrast, an abdominal X-ray gives a fetal radiation dose of 1.4 mGy, or an excess fatal childhood cancer risk of 1 in 24,000. Modern radiology departments can calculate the dose of radiation used in individual procedures if inadvertent exposure has occurred or determine the average amount applied in their department if a procedure is contemplated in pregnancy. The risk applies across the whole pregnancy, but is lower if it occurs in the first 6 weeks. Although exposure should always be minimized, if a procedure is likely to benefit the woman, in most cases the additional childhood cancer risk is unlikely on its own to be a reason to terminate the pregnancy.

(d) Fetal malformation, severe mental retardation and intrauterine death are the principal deterministic effects of external irradiation that can occur if the level of radiation is sufficiently high. In the first trimester, the minimal dose for fetal malformation is estimated at 500 mGy, which is equivalent to 360 abdominal X-rays (mean dose/procedure, 1.4 mGy), or 20 CT scans of the pelvis. There is the possibility of a non-threshold-type response in relation to mental retardation, interpreted as the loss of 30 intelligence quotient (IQ) points for each Gy of X-ray or gamma-ray exposure. However, even for a high-dose procedure, such as a CT scan of the pelvis, this represents, at most, the loss of <1 IQ point. In practice, radiation doses resulting from most diagnostic procedures do not present a substantial risk to an individual pregnancy.

(e) The risk of heritable disease is estimated at 1 in 42,000 per mGy exposure. This includes disease of varying severity, and so direct comparison with fatal cancer risks is unhelpful. However, the absolute risks are similar, although the consequences are potentially very different. An abdominal X-ray carries a risk of heritable disease of 1 in 30,000 and a CT scan of the pelvis has a risk of 1 in 1700. Because these risks are small, both absolutely and in comparison with background risks, inadvertent or unavoidable diagnostic procedures are not sufficient grounds alone to advise termination of a pregnancy.

1.33 PHENYLKETONURIA IN PREGNANCY

(a) The fundamental metabolic problem in phenylketonuria (PKU) is failure to metabolise tyrosine to phenylalanine.

(b) If the pregnant woman does not take the correct treatment, the risk to her child of severe intellectual handicap is over 90%.

(c) Fetal echocardiography should be offered to women with PKU in pregnancy.

(d) Breastfeeding is encouraged in most women.

(e) Pre-eclampsia is more common in women with PKU.

Answers

(a) F
(b) T
(c) T
(d) T
(e) F

Explanation

Ideally, women with PKU should have prepregnancy advice so that they conceive with phenylalanine levels as low as possible (target level, <0.6 mmol/l). This needs considerable encouragement and support, including expert dietetic input. In pregnancy, blood levels of phenylalanine should be measured at least every few weeks, which can usually be done at home using a capillary sample placed onto card and posted to the laboratory directly. Vomiting in early pregnancy and intercurrent infection must both be treated carefully and thoroughly because they could provoke a catabolic state in which the mother's own protein stores are broken down, increasing phenylalanine levels despite strict dietary compliance.

(a) PKU is an autosomal recessive condition in which 1 of 40 mutations in the phenylalanine hydroxylase gene results in inability to metabolise phenylalanine to tyrosine. In infancy, it is diagnosed by the Guthrie heel-prick test at the end of the first week of life. Phenylalanine is present is most natural proteins, which must therefore be withdrawn from the diet and replaced by an amino-acid substitute without phenylalanine. Failure to do so from birth to at least adolescence, when neurological development is complete, results in severe mental handicap.

(b) In pregnancy, a woman with PKU must take a strictly low-phenylalanine diet. Failure to do so results in increased circulating levels, which cross the placenta and cause irreversible intrauterine damage, including severe intellectual handicap in >90%, microcephaly in >70% and congenital heart disease, especially tetralogy of Fallot, in >10% of offspring.

(c) There is a significant risk of congenital heart defect.

(d) Assuming the baby does not have homozygous PKU similar to his/her mother, the risk of which is about 1% if the father's carrier status is unknown, breastfeeding should be encouraged. This is because the neonate has the metabolic capacity to deal with the extra phenylalanine load in the mother's milk.

(e) Pregnancy complications other than the adverse fetal effects outlined above are not more common than expected.

1.34 PSYCHIATRY

(a) In the UK, more women die from suicide than hypertensive disease of pregnancy.

(b) A women is five times more likely to commit suicide in the first 3 months postpartum than outside pregnancy.

(c) Suicide in pregnancy is less likely to be by violent means than outside pregnancy.
(d) A woman with a family history of bipolar disease has a one in three risk of puerperal psychosis.
(e) Puerperal psychosis affects 2 in 10,000 pregnancies.
(f) Most cases (95%) of puerperal psychosis occur in the first postnatal month.
(g) A woman with a history of puerperal psychosis has a 10% risk of recurrence after a future pregnancy.
(h) A woman with puerperal psychosis is more likely to be a professional or from a higher social class.

Answers

(a) T
(b) T
(c) F
(d) T
(e) F
(f) F
(g) F
(h) T

Explanation

(a) In the Confidential Enquiry into Maternal Deaths, 2000–02 [2], 60 women died from psychiatric causes and a further 28 women died from suicide; when the Office of National Statistics data are linked with childbirths in the preceding year, a further 42 and 32 cases, respectively, were identified. There were 14 hypertensive deaths in the same survey.
(b) The annual suicide rate is around 3.3 per 100,000 women, but the rate is five times higher in the postnatal period; if a woman has puerperal psychosis, her risk of suicide is 3 per 1000, which is 100 times greater than in the nonpregnant female population.
(c) Outside pregnancy, only around 20% of female suicides are violent; in pregnancy, almost 80% are violent deaths, which is the same as for male suicide.
(d) A family history of bipolar disease and a family history of puerperal psychosis are both very strong predictors of puerperal psychosis. Therefore, such histories should be sought, and appropriate management plans put in place.

(e) Puerperal psychosis affects 2 in 1000 pregnancies. Each unit should therefore have a robust relationship with their liaison psychiatrists.
(f) Of the total cases of puerperal psychosis, 50% of cases occur in the first 7 days after delivery, 75% of cases occur by day 16 and 95% of cases occur by day 90.
(g) If a woman has a history of puerperal psychosis, her risk of recurrence is 50%. The recurrence risk is also 50% if she has a history of schizophrenia, bipolar disorder, severe unipolar disorder or severe postnatal depression.
(h) Typically, women who suffer puerperal psychosis are professional women, including doctors, teachers, lawyers.

REFERENCES

1. Duley L, Henderson-Smart DJ, Knight M, King JF. Cochrane Pregnancy and Childbirth Group Antiplatelet agents for preventing pre-eclampsia and its complications. Cochrane Database of Systematic Reviews. 3, 2006.
2. Why Mothers Die 2000–02: Report on Confidential Enquiry into Maternal Deaths in the United Kingdom, 2004.
3. Cooper WO et al. Major congenital malformations after first trimester exposure to ACE inhibitors. *New Engl J Med* 2006; **354:** 2443–51.
4. Guidelines no55 @ www.sign.ac.uk/guidelines (accessed 13/10/6)
5. Confidential Enquiry into Maternal and Child Health, Pregnancy in Women with type 1 and type 2 diabetes, 2002–03 [2005].
6. Diabetes control and complication trial research group. The effect of intensive treatment of diabetes on the development of long-term complications in insulin dependent diabetes. *N Engl J Med* 1993; **329:** 977–86.
7. de Veciano M et al. Postprandial versus preprandial glucose monitoring in women with gestational diabetes mellitus requiring insulin therapy. *N Engl J Med* 1995; **333:** 1237–41.
8. Weiss PA et al. Long term follow up of infants of mothers with type 1 diabetes. Evidence for hereditary and nonhereditary transmission of diabetes and precursors. *Diabetes Care* 2000; **23:** 905–11.
9. Medical eligibility criteria for contraceptive use, 3rd edn (2004). http://www.who.int (accessed 10/10/06)
10. The British Eclampsia Survey Douglas KA, Redman CW. Eclampsia in the United Kingdom. *Br Med J* 1994; **309:** 139–400.

11. Haddow JE et al. Maternal thyroid deficiency during pregnancy and subsequent neuropsychological development of the child. *N Engl J Med* 1999; **341:** 549–55.

12. Lazarus J. Guidelines for the Use of Radioiodine in the Management of Hyperthyroidism: A Summary Prepared by the Radioiodine Audit Subcommittee of the Royal College of Physicians on Diabetes and Endocrinology and the Research Unit of the Royal College of Physicians. *J R Coll Physicians Lond* 1995; **29:** 464–69.

13. Momotani N et al. Maternal hyperthyroidism and congenital malformation in the offspring. *Clin Endocrin* 1984; **20:** 695–700.

14. Othman S et al. A long term follow up of postpartum thyroiditis. *Clin Endocrinol* 1990; **32:** 559–64.

15. Lazarus JH et al. Clinical aspects of recurrent postpartum thyroiditis. *Br J Gen Pract* 1997; **47:** 305–08.

16. Van den Broe NR and Letsky EA. Pregnancy and the erythrocyte sedimentation rate. *Br J Obstet Gynaecol* 2001; **108:** 1164–7.

17. Kothari A et al. Tuberculosis and pregnancy – results of a study in a high prevalence area of London. *Eur J Obstet Gynaecol and Repod Biol* 2006; **126:** 48–55.

18. Making the best use of a Department of Clinical Radiology, Guidelines for Doctors, 3rd edn. The Royal College of Radiologists, London; 1995.

Chapter 2
Extended Matching Questions

2.1 HYPERTENSION

The following women have all presented with hypertension in pregnancy. Choose the most likely diagnosis from the list below:

(a) Phaeochromocytoma
(b) Pregnancy-induced hypertension
(c) Reflux nephropathy
(d) Cushing's syndrome
(e) Pre-eclampsia
(f) Conn's syndrome
(g) Renal artery stenosis
(h) Coarctation of the aorta
(i) Systemic lupus erythematosus (SLE)
(j) Essential hypertension

1. At 11 weeks' gestation, a 34 year old primiparous woman is found to have a booking blood pressure of 126/74 mmHg and normal urinalysis. At 39 weeks' gestation, she is found to have a blood pressure of 144/96 mmHg; urinalysis shows trace proteinuria and 1+ glycosuria.

2. At 11 weeks' gestation, a 22 year old primiparous woman is found to have a booking blood pressure of 164/102 mmHg and normal urinalysis. Serum creatinine is 66 μmol/l and serum potassium is 3.2 mmol/l.

3. At 11 weeks' gestation, a 30 year old primiparous woman is found to have a booking blood pressure of 152/94 mmHg and urinalysis shows 2+ protein and 3+ blood. Serum creatinine is 159 μmol/l and serum potassium is 4.6 mmol/l.

4. At 11 weeks' gestation, a 29 year old primiparous woman is found to have a booking blood pressure of 132/76 mmHg and normal urinalysis. At 35 weeks' gestation, she is found to have a blood pressure of 154/98 mmHg; urinalysis shows 2+ proteinuria.

5. At 11 weeks' gestation, a 19 year old primiparous woman is found to have a booking blood pressure of 160/104 mmHg and urinalysis shows 3+ protein. Serum creatinine is 132 μmol/l and serum potassium is 4.1 mmol/l.

Answers

1. (b)
2. (f)
3. (i)
4. (e)
5. (c)

Explanation

1. New-onset hypertension in the late third trimester in the absence of significant proteinuria is most likely to be pregnancy-induced hypertension. In pregnancy, 1+ glycosuria is common and nonpathological.
2. Pre-existing hypertension with co-incident hypokalaemia suggests an underlying diagnosis of hyperaldosteronism.
3. Pre-existing hypertension with renal impairment and both haematuria and proteinuria points to a diagnosis of underlying renal disease. Haematuria would favour a diagnosis of SLE.
4. New-onset hypertension in the third trimester with new-onset proteinuria is most likely to be pre-eclampsia.
5. Pre-existing hypertension with renal impairment and proteinuria points to a diagnosis of underlying renal disease. This is most likely to be because of reflux nephropathy. SLE is also possible.

2.2 HEART SOUNDS AND MURMURS

The following women are all found to have a heart murmur or added sound. Choose the most likely auscultatory abnormality from the list below:

(a) Early diastolic murmur
(b) Mid-systolic click
(c) Ejection systolic murmur
(d) Pan-systolic murmur
(e) Late-systolic murmur
(f) Third heart sound
(g) Opening snap

(h) Venous hum
(i) Mid-diastolic murmur
(j) Fourth heart sound

1. A Somalian primiparous woman at 27 weeks' gestation presents to an obstetric day assessment unit with orthopnoea.
2. A multiparous woman on an obstetric high-dependency unit, who presented with breathlessness 2 weeks after delivery by Caesarean section. Echocardiogram confirms the diagnosis of peripartum cardiomyopathy.
3. A 30 year old primiparous woman with a bioprosthetic aortic-valve replacement 20 years previously presents with breathlessness at 30 weeks' gestation.
4. A 33 year old American is referred at 16 weeks' gestation with a history of palpitations. She brings the results of previous investigations, which include an echocardiogram showing posterior movement of one mitral valve cusp during systole.
5. A 20 year old woman with hypertension discovered at booking at 14 weeks' gestation is found to have radiofemoral delay.

Answers

1. (i)
2. (d) or (f)
3. (a)
4. (b)
5. (e)

Explanation

1. Orthopnoea because of pulmonary oedema in an immigrant with mitral stenosis secondary to rheumatic fever. Pulmonary oedema has been precipitated by the increased cardiac output and tachycardia at this gestation. An opening snap might also be heard.
2. Peripartum cardiomyopathy is a dilated cardiomyopathy leading to, in this case, mitral regurgitation, causing a pan-systolic murmur and a gallup rhythm or third heart sound.
3. This is aortic regurgitation because of a failing prosthetic heart valve.
4. This is mitral valve prolapse.
5. This is coarctation of the aorta that could cause a mid-to-late systolic murmur.

2.3 ANAEMIA

The following women have presented with anaemia. Please choose
the most appropriate cause of their anaemia.

(a) Autoimmune haemolytic anaemia because of SLE
(b) Autoimmune haemolytic anaemia (AIHA) because of methyldopa administration
(c) HELLP syndrome
(d) Blood loss
(e) Iron deficiency
(f) Sickle cell disease
(g) Coeliac disease
(h) Hereditary spherocytosis
(i) Alpha thalassaemia trait
(j) Pernicious anaemia

1. A 38 year old multiparous woman with hypothyroidism presents with dyspepsia and shortness of breath on exercise at 30
   weeks' gestation. She has a megaloblastic anaemia and parietal
   cell antibodies.
2. A 24 year old multiparous woman with a 1-year history of
   abdominal pain and steatorrhoea is found to have a booking
   haemoglobin (Hb) concentration of 9.1 g/dl, high MCV and normal MCHC. A blood film shows hypersegmented neutrophils.
3. An 18 year old primiparous woman presents at 23 weeks' gestation with a Hb concentration of 9.3 g/dl, low MCV, low MCHC
   and platelet count of 540×10^9 platelets/l.
4. A 40 year old multiparous woman presents at 33 weeks' gestation
   with hypertension and abdominal pain. She is found to be anaemic,
   with a Hb concentration of 8.9 g/dl, normal MCV and normal
   MCHC 5 days after admission. A blood film shows spherocytes,
   her reticulocyte count is high and a Coombs' test is positive.
5. An 18 year old primiparous woman presents at 23 weeks' gestation
   with a Hb concentration of 9.3 g/dl, low MCV, normal MCHC
   and platelet count of 234×10^9 platelets/l.

Answers

1. (j)
2. (g)
3. (d)
4. (b)
5. (i)

Explanation

1. Megaloblastic anaemia because of a failure of absorption of vitamin B12 and consequent vitamin B12 deficiency because of pernicious anaemia. Autoimmune gastritis leads to destruction of parietal cells and lack of intrinsic factor, which is essential for vitamin B12 absorption. Pernicious anaemia is associated with atrophic autoimmune hypothyroidism.

2. Macrocytic normochromic anaemia. Megaloblastic anaemia because of a failure of absorption of folate due to coeliac disease. Hypersegmented neutrophils are characteristic in the peripheral blood in megaloblastic anaemia. Bone marrow aspiration would show megaloblasts (large erythroblasts with immature nuclei).

3. This woman has a microcytic hypochromic anaemia, of which the commonest cause would be iron deficiency. However, the raised platelet count suggests recent blood loss.

4. This woman has a normocytic normochromic anaemia. The presence of spherocytes in the blood film support a diagnosis of haemolytic anaemia. The direct antiglobulin test (DAT; Coombs' test) detects autoantibodies on the surface of the red blood cells and, if positive, indicates an autoimmune haemolytic anaemia. In hereditary spherocytosis, Coombs' test is negative and the osmotic fragility test is positive. Methyldopa is a well-recognised cause of AIHA and is a common drug choice for treatment of hypertension in pregnancy.

5. This woman has a microcytic normochromic anaemia, making an alpha thalassaemia trait a more likely diagnosis than iron deficiency (when all the indices are reduced). These individuals are normally asymptomatic but could become anaemic during pregnancy, in which case they should receive iron and folate supplements.

2.4 CHEST PAIN

A pregnant woman has "chest pain". Match the following clinical scenarios to the diagnoses below:

(a) Pulmonary embolus
(b) Myocardial infarction
(c) Pneumonia
(d) Tietze's syndrome
(e) Rib fracture
(f) Reflux oesophagitis
(g) Angina
(h) Amniotic fluid embolus

(i) Tuberculosis (TB)

(j) Pneumothorax

1. A 40 year old woman at term in uncomplicated labour suddenly becomes dyspnoeic and develops central chest pain before collapsing; during the resuscitation, you notice extensive bruising.

2. A 40 year old woman at term in uncomplicated labour suddenly becomes dyspnoeic and develops central chest pain before collapsing; during the resuscitation, you are told that she has been hypertensive for several years.

3. A 40 year old woman at term in uncomplicated labour suddenly becomes dyspnoeic and develops central chest pain before collapsing; during the resuscitation, you notice that she has Q-waves in lead III of the electrocardiogram (ECG).

4. On chest examination, the trachea is central, there is dullness to percussion and whispering pectoriloquy.

5. On chest examination, the trachea is deviated to the left and, at the left apex, there is dullness to percussion and whispering pectoriloquy.

6. On chest examination, the trachea is deviated to the right and there is reduced air entry on the left, with hyper-resonance on percussion.

7. On chest examination, there is tenderness when the thorax is compressed.

8. On chest examination, there is tenderness over the costochondral margins.

Answers

1. (h)
2. (b)
3. (a)
4. (c)
5. (i)
6. (j)
7. (e)
8. (d)

Explanation

1. Amniotic fluid embolus is a rare complication of pregnancy, typically occurring during otherwise uncomplicated labour. If fetal squames are found in central blood or maternal sputum, this supports the diagnosis. Typically, the presentation is sudden collapse requiring resuscitation; the condition has a high mortality

rate. DIC is a common complication, and could reveal itself as bruising or bleeding.

2. Although myocardial infarction is rare in pregnancy, its frequency is gradually increasing, as more women with risk factors for cardiovascular disease become pregnant. During pregnancy, the extra work of the heart increases markedly in the first trimester and then again in labour. Once the diagnosis has been considered, it can be confirmed by measuring blood troponin levels, ECG changes and cardiac enzyme changes, which evolve in the normal way.

3. Pulmonary embolism is the leading direct cause of maternal mortality in the UK and should always be considered when a pregnant woman collapses. The classic ECG changes of an S-wave in lead I and a Q-wave plus inverted T-wave in lead III of the ECG are nonspecific and can occur in normal pregnancy.

4. When examining the respiratory system, the trachea must be palpated to establish whether it is pulled towards an area of fibrosis or scarring, or deviated away from a large pneumothorax or pleural effusion. Asymmetry of chest-wall expansion can also give a clue to the site of the pathology, in addition to percussion, which will be dull in consolidation, stony dull in pleural effusion and might be hyper-resonant in pneumothorax. Air entry might be reduced if there is a large pneumothorax or effusion. Tactile vocal fremitus (the ability to feel sounds vibrating through to the chest wall with a hand laid flat, palm downwards, on the chest) and whispering pectoriloquy (whispered sounds heard distinctly through a stethoscope held over the area of pathology) occur with pneumonia and fibrosis. These findings are typical of pneumonia.

5. TB typical affects the apices of the lung and causes fibrosis which draws the trachea across towards the affected side.

6. These findings are typical of pneumothorax.

7. Localized pain on chest wall compression suggests the possibility of rib fracture.

8. Tietze's syndrome is also known as "costochondritis" and results from inflammation in the cartilage that joins rib to sternum.

2.5 CAUSES OF ADRENAL DYSFUNCTION

From the causes of adrenal dysfunction listed below, choose the most appropriate diagnosis in the following clinical scenarios:

(a) Addison's disease
(b) Conn's syndrome
(c) Pituitary Cushing's syndrome
(d) Adrenal carcinoma

(e) Lymphocytic hypophysitis
(f) Sheehan's syndrome
(g) Phaeochromocytoma
(h) Exogenous steroid therapy adrenal suppression
(i) Radiotherapy
(j) Congenital adrenal hyperplasia

1. A 32 year old women presents to the infertility clinic with a history
    of secondary infertility and amenorrhoea. She describes lethargy
    and loss of libido. On closer questioning, she admits to symptoms
    of depression following failure to breastfeed her first child who was
    born by emergency Caesarean section 13 months previously.

2. A 30 year old primiparous woman attends Day Assessment Unit
    (DAU) at 28 weeks' gestation because she has been experiencing
    daily palpitations for 3 months. These are accompanied by
    extreme anxiety. Her booking blood pressure at 11 weeks' gesta-
    tion was 138/94 mmHg. She has no family history of hypertension.
    Her blood pressure on admission to the DAU is 124/68 mmHg but
    during the CTG recording (10 minutes later) her blood pressure is
    documented as 158/102 mmHg.

3. A 23 year old women with brittle asthma complains of dizziness
    3 hours after a normal vaginal delivery with minimal blood loss.
    You review her on the postnatal ward and find her blood pressure
    to be 84/53 mmHg. Her heart rate is 76 bpm, lochia is normal
    and her Hb concentration is 11.5 g/dl.

4. A 36 year old multiparous woman book for antenatal care at 14
    weeks' gestation. You find her blood pressure to be 154/98 mmHg;
    she has 3+ glycosuria, a body mass index of 38 and you notice
    bruises on all four limbs and marked, purple abdominal striae. Her
    ACTH level, requested by the endocrine registrar 1 week previ-
    ously, is below the normal range for a nonpregnant woman.

5. A 28 year old women with type 1 diabetes mellitus collapses 12
    hours following a ventouse delivery at 39 weeks' gestation. Her
    blood pressure is 88/60 mmHg, her Hb concentration is
    13.1 g/dl, serum sodium level is 132 mmol/l, serum potassium is
    5.3 mmol/l and blood glucose is 3.3 mmol/l. Following delivery,
    her insulin sliding scale was adjusted to half the rate of insulin
    compared with labour and was discontinued following breakfast
    1 hour before the collapse. She has received no insulin since.

Answers

1. (f)
2. (g)
3. (h)

4. (d)
5. (a)

Explanation

1. Sheehan's syndrome classically presents as a failure to lactate. It is caused by pituitary infarction following postpartum haemorrhage. Subsequent features include a failure to resume menstruation, loss of secondary sexual characteristics, hypothyroidism (where the thyroid stimulating hormone (TSH) is inappropriately low despite reduced free low fT_4 level) and adrenal insufficiency.

2. Phaeochromocytoma could present with fluctuating or labile hypertension, and hypertension might occur in the supine position because of the pressure of the gravid uterus on the tumour. Tachycardia and anxiety are caused by the intermittent secretion of catecholamines from the tumour.

3. Endogenous production of corticosteroids from the adrenal glands is suppressed if exogenous steroids are given in high doses for prolonged periods of time. This woman with brittle asthma was receiving prednisolone (30 mg/day) for most of her pregnancy but no supplementary parenteral steroids were given to cover the stress of her labour, and because she arrived on the post natal ward at 10 a.m., she has missed the morning drug round. Women taking oral steroids should be given intravenous hydrocortisone 50 mg 6 hourly from the onset of labour until 24 hours after delivery.

4. This woman has typical features of Cushing's syndrome. This is more likely to be because of adrenal, rather than pituitary, causes in pregnancy. An adrenal cause is confirmed by the low ACTH level, which is suppressed because of excess corticosteroid production by the adrenal tumour. Pituitary Cushing's syndrome would be more likely if the ACTH level was high (although levels are higher in any case during pregnancy because of placental production).

5. Addison's disease because of autoimmune destruction of the adrenal glands is more common in women with type I diabetes. This woman has collapsed because of mineralocorticoid insufficiency, which is probably compounded by the relative volume depletion of labour and delivery. She was on a sliding scale, and was likely to be receiving intravenous 5% or 10% dextrose solution rather than saline, further exacerbating sodium depletion. Her blood glucose level is low, despite receiving no insulin, because insulin requirements are reduced with corticosteroid insufficiency. Her blood glucose is, however, not low enough to explain the collapse.

2.6 CONNECTIVE TISSUE DISEASE

Consider the following connective tissue disorders and match them with the most appropriate clinical scenario from the list below:

(a) Sarcoid
(b) SLE
(c) APS
(d) Rheumatoid arthritis
(e) Normal pregnancy
(f) Sjogren's syndrome
(g) TB
(h) Ankylosing spondylitis
(i) Osteoarthritis

1. At booking, a 35 year old woman gives a history of haematuria and proteinuria. She also has a past medical history of photosensitive facial erythema and arthralgia.
2. A 25 year old pregnant woman presents with dyspnoea. She has a normal chest X-ray, normal oxygen saturation and raised ACE levels.
3. At booking a 39 year old gives a history of stiff joints in her hands, which fluctuates and often completely resolves; she is also found to have a mild normocytic anaemia.
4. A 22 year old woman's first baby is born with a facial rash that resolves after a few months. The paediatricians question the mother and discover that she has dry mouth and gritty eyes.
5. A 40 year old pregnant woman presents with dyspnoea and painful red eyes; she has a restrictive lung picture, with reduced transfer factor and granulomata on pleural biopsy.
6. A 29 year old with a history of bloody diarrhoea and abdominal pain develops a stiff lower back during pregnancy.

Answers

1. (b)
2. (e)
3. (d)
4. (f)
5. (a)
6. (h)

Explanation

1. This lady has SLE. Butterfly rash and photosensitivity are typical of SLE, which can manifest as abnormalities in every body system,

and frequently also includes nonspecific symptoms, such as fatigue and fever. It is nine times more common in women than men, and is especially prevalent in black women, affecting 1 in 250. Women with SLE need close surveillance in pregnancy, especially if their disease is active. Those women with hypertension or renal involvement have an increased risk of pre-eclampsia; they should have antiphospholipid antibodies and the extractable nuclear antigens, anti-Ro and anti-La measured (see below), because these might have a direct bearing on the pregnancy outcome.

2. These can each be features in a normal pregnancy. The subjective feeling of dyspnoea is common in pregnancy. Usually, the absence of any associated clinical features (cardiovascular or respiratory) and the clear onset of symptoms during the pregnancy should enable appropriate reassurance. Some groups of women, especially those recently arrived from overseas, have a higher risk of a variety of medical problems (including congenital and rheumatic heart disease and TB) and might warrant a lower threshold for investigation of dyspnoea in pregnancy. Depending on the clinical scenario, it might be appropriate to perform a chest X-ray, an ECG, arterial blood gases, etc. Serum ACE levels are helpful in the diagnosis of sarcoidosis outside pregnancy, but are rarely measured after conception because they are frequently raised in normal pregnancy.

3. Rheumatoid arthritis most commonly occurs in women aged between 30 and 50 years and follows a relapsing and remitting course. Typically, the small joints of the hand are painful and stiff, especially in the morning, and appear warm, tender and swollen. There is often associated malaise and some extra-articular involvement. Seropositivity for rheumatoid factor is found in 70% of these patients.

4. The facial rash is neonatal cutaneous lupus, which occurs in 5% of the babies whose mothers are anti-Ro or anti-La positive: 2% of such women will have a fetus with congenital heart block, which could manifest in utero as fetal bradycardia, hydrops fetalis or intrauterine death. Treatment has limited success, but may include steroids and plasmapheresis; ultimately, delivery is required, although the neonate could require long-term pacing. In both cases, the risk of recurrence in a subsequent pregnancy is around 16–44%. Anti-Ro and anti-La can occasionally occur in asymptomatic women. More commonly there is an associated connective tissue disorder: they occur in 70% of women with Sjogren's syndrome and 10% of women with rheumatoid arthritis and SLE. In this case, the diagnosis is Sjogren's syndrome.

5. This lady has sarcoidosis. The major causes of granulomata in lung tissue are TB and sarcoidosis, the former causing cavitating lesions. The other respiratory findings in sarcoidosis include

bihilar lymphadenopathy, widespread ground glass shadowing, restrictive lung defect and pulmonary hypertension. On lung function testing, this patient would have a decreased total lung capacity, reduction in both FEV1 and FVC, and decreased gas transfer. The latter might be useful for early diagnosis and assessment of progression of diseases of the lung parenchyma, such as pulmonary fibrosis, asbestosis and sarcoidosis.

6. Ankylosing spondylitis is associated with inflammatory bowel disease, which is the likely diagnosis here. Although isolated ankylosing spondylitis is much more common in men than women, this is not true when it is associated with other conditions. This woman needs investigation of her gastrointestinal symptoms.

2.7 LIVER DISEASE

From the causes of abnormal liver function tests (LFT) listed below, choose the most appropriate diagnosis to fit the following clinical scenarios:

(a) Acute fatty liver of pregnancy (AFLP)
(b) Obstetric cholestasis (OC)
(c) HELLP syndrome
(d) Acute hepatitis A
(e) Chronic hepatitis B
(f) Dubin–Johnson syndrome
(g) Drug reaction
(h) Acute cholecystitis
(i) Crigler–Najjar syndrome
(j) Liver haematoma
(k) Normal pregnancy
(l) Post-Caesarean section
(m) Primary biliary cirrhosis (PBC)
(n) Nonalcoholic steatohepatitis (NASH)
(o) Gilbert's syndrome
(p) Haemolysis
(q) Pre-eclampsia
(r) Sclerosing cholangitis

Mrs X is at 35 weeks' gestation. She presents with RUQ pain, fever, nausea and malaise. Her blood pressure is 140/90 mmHg and her urine shows 1+ proteinuria.

1. Her temperature is 37.6°C, ALT is 300 iu/ml, WBC is $28 \times 10^9/l$, urate is 692 µmol/l, RBG is 3.6 mmol/l and platelet count is $153 \times 10^9/l$.

2. Her temperature is 39.3°C, ALT is 60 iu/ml, WBC is $21 \times 10^9/l$, urate is 350 µmol/l, RBG is 6.8 mmol/l and platelet count is $221 \times 10^9/l$.

3. Her temperature is 37.2°C, ALT is 60 iu/ml, WBC is $12 \times 10^9/l$, urate is 400 μmol/l, RBG is 5.3 mmol/l and platelet count is 100.

Mrs Y is has not booked and is around 32 weeks' gestation. She presents with pruritus, malaise and reduced fetal movements. Her ALT is 250 iu/ml.

4. Her ultrasound shows a small, fibrotic liver.
5. Her liver ultrasound shows diffuse architectural change, and on liver biopsy, portal tract infiltration and granulomata are observed.
6. Her liver ultrasound is normal.

Mrs W has had an upper respiratory tract infection, which was treated by her GP. She makes a good recovery, and shortly after, attends an antenatal clinic. At the clinic, she is thought by her midwife to look yellow, so LFTs are performed.

7. Her bilirubin is 32 μmol/l, ALT is 270 iu/ml and urine dipstick bilinogen large.
8. Her bilirubin is 10 μmol/l, ALT is 23 iu/ml and urine dipstick small urobilinogen.
9. Her bilirubin is 51 μmol/l (unconjugated, 47 μmol/l and conjugated, 4 μmol/l), ALT is 19 iu/ml and urine large urobilinogen.

Mrs Z attends your obstetric medicine clinic with the following:

10. An episode of bloody, painful diarrhoea, and she is found to have a significantly raised alkaline phosphatase (>1000 iu/l).
11. Type 2 diabetes, obesity and raised gamma-glutamyl transferase (70 iu/l).
12. Hereditary spherocytosis, and you also find that her bilirubin is 35 μmol/l.

Answers

1. (a)
2. (h)
3. (c)
4. (e)
5. (m)
6. (b)
7. (g)
8. (k)
9. (o)
10. (r)
11. (n)
12. (p)

Explanation

There is a broad differential diagnosis if abnormal LFTs are encountered in pregnancy. It is important to remember that the reference range quoted by the laboratory for transaminases, bilirubin and gamma-glutamyl transferase are approximately 20% lower and alkaline phosphatase up to three times greater in pregnancy than outside pregnancy [1]. After delivery, LFTs return to the nonpregnant range, but could initially increase substantially in the first few days, especially if delivery is by Caesarean section [2].

Mrs X represents a typical, and possibly confusing, presentation in late pregnancy.

1. AFLP often presents as a nonspecific illness with low-grade temperature, marked leucocytosis and hyperuricaemia beyond that which is usually seen in pre-eclampsia. Blood pressure and urinary protein levels might suggest pre-eclampsia, but the degree of abnormality of the LFTs is usually out of keeping with the apparently mild pre-eclampsia. Typically, LFTs deteriorate rapidly, so whenever the diagnosis is considered, LFTs should be repeated after 6 hours. Unlike other forms of pregnancy-specific liver dysfunction (i.e. HELLP syndrome, pre-eclampsia obesteric cholestasis and hyperemesis gravidarum), liver failure might develop with hypoglycaemia, because of the inability of the liver to store glycogen, and a coagulopathy, because of impaired hepatic production of clotting factors, especially factor II (prothrombin), which has the shortest half-life of all the coagulation factors. AFLP is best treated by prompt delivery. If there is no obvious and sustained improvement in liver function, transfer the patient to a hepatic intensive care unit for specialist liver support and consideration of urgent liver transplantation.

2. Acute cholecystitis can present at any gestation of pregnancy. Typically, there is severe right upper quadrant pain, with fever, systemic upset and tenderness, especially on inspiration, in the right hypochondrium. There could be history of intolerance to fatty foods, which in pregnancy might be confused with heartburn secondary to hormone-induced incompetence of the oesophageal sphincter. The diagnosis is supported by significant fever, bacteraemia, thickening of the gallbladder wall on ultrasound, usually with gallstone(s), and a dilated biliary tract. Near-term management is usually supportive, with analgesia, antibiotics and control of fever. Although cholecystectomy can be carried out in pregnancy, it is best delayed until after the acute episode, and unless remote from term, until after delivery.

3. HELLP syndrome typically presents near term or in the early puerperium with right upper quadrant pain secondary to liver capsule oedema, pre-eclampsia, which seems mild, and the biochemical

parameters that fulfil the acronym (as described above). The main-stay of treatment is delivery for the antenatal patient, combined with supportive management. There is some evidence that steroids might ameliorate the course of the disease. These can be considered in unusual cases that continue to deteriorate postpartum [3, 4].

Patients who have not been booked are more likely to have sig-nificant obstetric and/or medical problems than women who booked in the first trimester.

4. This scenario is chronic hepatitis B carriage with cirrhosis. She needs to have blood taken to assess her e-antigen status and viral load. Lamivudine might be of value for reducing her chance of pro-gressing to end-stage liver failure. Her baby needs vaccination against hepatitis B at delivery and gamma-globulin if she is a high infectivity carrier. Her partner must have his hepatitis B status checked. Depending on the likely route of transmission, she needs to be tested for other viral infections, including hepatitis C and human immunodeficiency virus (HIV). She needs referral to a hepatologist.

5. Primary biliary cirrhosis is 10 times more common in women than men, and typically presents in the fourth or fifth decade of life with pruritus and abnormal LFTs, especially a raised alkaline phos-phatase level. The diagnosis is established by finding antimito-chondrial antibodies, which should be measured in every pregnant woman with unexplained itching and elevated liver enzymes. Liver biopsy, which may be deferred until after delivery, will typically demonstrate granulomata.

6. Obstetric cholestasis occurs in around 1 in 160 pregnancies. Typical symptoms are pruritus, often with general tiredness or malaise. It is a diagnosis of exclusion. Therefore, in addition to the normal ultrasound, she needs a viral and autoimmune screen.

7. Drug reactions are a common cause of abnormal LFTs. Co-amoxiclav is one of the commonest causes. It is important to identify the drug responsible and discontinue it: usually the LFTs will then return to normal range.

8. This is normal. Clearly, the midwife was mistaken in her concern about "looking yellow".

9. Gilbert's syndrome is a benign, familial cause of unconjugated hyperbilirubinaemia, which affects up to 7% of the population. It is due to reduced levels of the hepatocyte membrane enzyme that takes up unconjugated bilirubin and conjugates it (thereby ren-dering it water-soluble). Fasting, intercurrent infection and preg-nancy can each cause bilirubin levels to increase, and could result in clinically apparent jaundice. The unconjugated fraction of bilirubin is over 90% of the total bilirubin, and other LFTs are

normal. The reticulocyte count is normal, excluding haemolysis. The condition is benign and does not usually warrant further investigation. Treatment is only of the precipitating factor.

10. This patient has inflammatory bowel disease, most likely ulcerative colitis (UC). The raised alkaline phosphatase level is because of primary sclerosing cholangitis (PSC), a chronic fibrosing liver disease, with inflammatory destruction of bile ducts. Of people with sclerosing cholangitis, 75% have UC; 2.5–7.5% people with ulcerative colitis develop PSC.

11. NASH is common in obese individuals, and might form part of the spectrum of insulin-resistant conditions or the metabolic syndrome. Its presentation is very different from, and it is not related to, AFLP.

12. Hereditary spherocytosis is an autosomal dominant cause of haemolytic anaemia, affecting 1 in 5000 northern Europeans. Typically, the blood film shows spherocytes and reticulocytes, and anaemia might also be present. The direct Coombs' test is negative, thereby excluding autoimmune haemolysis. Bilirubin is predominantly unconjugated, and is raised because of the breakdown of haemoglobin in excess of the liver uptake mechanisms.

REFERENCES

1. Girling JC, Dow E, and Smith JH. Liver function tests in preeclampsia: The importance of comparison with a reference range derived for normal pregnancy. *Br J Obstet Gynaecol* 1997; **104:** 246–50.

2. David A, Kotecha M, and Girling JC. Factors influencing postnatal liver function tests. *Br J Obstet Gynaecol* 2000; **107:** 1421–26.

3. Magann EF, Perry KG Jr, Meydrech EF, Harris RL, Chauhan SP, Martin JN Jr. Postpartum corticosteroids: accelerated recovery from the syndrome of hemolysis, elevated liver enzymes, and low platelets (HELLP). Clinical Trial. Journal Article. *American Journal of Obstetrics & Gynecology* 1994; **171:** 1154–8.

4. Magann EF, Bass D, Chauhan SP, Sullivan DL, Martin RW, Martin JN Jr. Antepartum corticosteroids: disease stabilization in patients with the syndrome of hemolysis, elevated liver enzymes, and low platelets (HELLP). *American Journal of Obstetrics & Gynecology* 1994; **171:** 1148–53.

Chapter 3
Short Answer Questions/Data Interpretation/Clinical Scenarios

3.1 HYPERTENSION AND PROTEINURIA

You are asked to review a 39 year old woman on the antenatal ward. She is 33 weeks into her first ongoing pregnancy. She suffered a miscarriage at 9 weeks' gestation in her first pregnancy 2 years ago. She booked with a blood pressure of 136/78 mmHg and urinalysis was negative. Her antenatal course has been uneventful and she had a normal anomaly scan at 20 weeks. She was admitted from the antenatal clinic 3 days ago because she was found to have 1+ proteinuria and her blood pressure was 148/96 mmHg. Since admission, her blood pressure has ranged from 132–154 mmHg systolic and 86–104 mmHg diastolic. She has received no treatment since admission. Blood tests performed on admission revealed the following results:

Haemoglobin (Hb): 13.1 g/dl
Platelet: 152×10^9/l
Creatinine: 86 µmol/l
ALT: 23 iu/l
AlkP: 210 iu/l
Bilirubin: 9 µmol/l
Albumin: 25 g/l
Uric acid: 0.39 mmol/l

The midwife is concerned because the 24-hour urine collection result has come back as 6.2 g protein/24 hours.

1. What is the diagnosis?
2. What other investigations would you arrange?
3. What treatment would you give?
4. What would you tell the woman?

Answers

1. The diagnosis is pre-eclampsia. This woman has new-onset hypertension and significant proteinuria. The diagnosis is further

supported by relatively high haemoglobin, suggesting haemoconcentration, uric acid that is above the normal range for 33 weeks' gestation and serum creatinine that is also higher than expected at 33 weeks' gestation.

2. Other appropriate investigations would include an ultrasound scan of the fetus to assess fetal growth and liquor volume, umbilical Doppler/regular CTGs to monitor fetal well-being, serial blood tests to monitor platelet count, renal function and serum albumin, and liver function tests. At 33 weeks' gestation, minor abnormalities in blood chemistry might prompt delivery, for example:

Platelet: $<100 \times 10^9/l$
Serum albumin: <20 g/l
ALT/AST: above the normal range for pregnancy
Creatinine: >100 μmol/l

3. Whether to treat this (moderate) level of hypertension in pregnancy is controversial. A blood pressure above 170/110 mmHg should definitely be treated, but there is no evidence that lower levels are immediately harmful to the mother, and overzealous control of blood pressure could risk jeopardizing uteroplacental perfusion and the fetus. Treating blood pressure will reduce the risk of episodes of severe hypertension that could be harmful or lead to delivery that would not otherwise be indicated. On balance, begin treatment with methyldopa, 250 mg three times daily. The Royal College of Obstetricians and Gynaecologists (RCOG) [1] guidelines also recommend the use of antenatal steroids to induce fetal lung maturation at gestations of up to 34–36 weeks. Therefore, also prescribe two doses of betamethasone, 12 mg 12 hours apart. Because of the risks of age (39 years), nephrotic range proteinuria, pre-eclampsia and relative immobility in hospital, thromboprophylaxis with thromboembolic deterrent stockings and low molecular weight heparin (e.g. enoxaparin, 40 mg subcutaneously daily) should be commenced.

4. The woman should be informed of the diagnosis; explain pre-eclampsia to her. She should be advised to remain in hospital until delivery and that delivery is likely to be required within the next 2–3 weeks. The rationale for antenatal steroids, thromboprophylaxis and antihypertensives should be explained and the plan for monitoring both her and her baby discussed. She should be informed of the "symptoms" of pre-eclampsia (headache and epigastric pain) and placental abruption (vaginal bleeding and abdominal pain) and advised to inform a midwife or doctor if she experiences these or any reduction in fetal movements. She should be offered counselling from a neonatologist and a visit to the neonatal unit. She has an increased risk of delivery by Caesaeran section, so this should be discussed and an anaesthetic review arranged.

3.2 HYPERTENSION AND PROTEINURIA

A 24 year old multiparous woman is admitted to the antenatal ward at 29 weeks' gestation with a blood pressure of 152/92 mmHg and 4+ proteinuria. She is asymptomatic apart from oedema affecting her fingers, face and legs. An ultrasound scan reveals a normally grown fetus and normal liquor volume. Her booking blood pressure was 104/68 mmHg and urinalysis at 11 weeks' gestation was negative. Blood tests on admission show the following:

Hb:	12.4 g/l
WBC:	$5.1 \times 10^9/l$
Platelet:	$175 \times 10^9/l$
Uric acid:	0.33 mmol/l
Urea:	4.2 mmol/l
Creatinine:	77 μmol/l
ALT:	23 iu/l
Albumin:	25 g/l

A 24-hour urine collection reveals 6.5 g of protein. She receives two doses of betamethasone, 12 g intramuscularly and is treated with methyldopa 500 mg three times daily. After one week, her blood pressure is 130–140/84–96 mmHg. She remains asymptomatic and blood chemistry results are as follows:

Hb:	11.3 g/l
WBC:	$17.2 \times 10^9/l$
Platelet:	$140 \times 10^9/l$
Uric acid:	0.35 mmol/l
Urea:	6.4 mmol/l
Creatinine:	87 μmol/l
ALT:	28 iu/l
Albumin:	22 g/l

A repeat 24-hour urine collection shows 13.9 g of protein.

1. What is the likely cause of leucocytosis?
2. Do you think this women needs to be delivered? Explain your answer.

Answers

1. This patient has new-onset hypertension and proteinuria. The diagnosis is pre-eclampsia, which is supported by the relative haemoconcentration, a uric acid level that is high for this gestation, a falling platelet count and a rising creatinine. Although not abnormal outside pregnancy, a serum creatinine of 87 μmol/l is

above the normal limit for the third trimester of pregnancy (normal, 70–75 μmol/l).

The patient has been appropriately admitted to hospital, but her fetus is well grown, her blood pressure is well controlled on methyldopa and she is asymptomatic. Leucocytosis is likely to be due to betamethasone therapy. At this gestation, every effort should be made to prolong the pregnancy and gain fetal maturity. Although she has heavy proteinuria, this in itself is not an indication for delivery. With this degree of proteinuria, she is likely to become more hypoalbuminaemic.

2. Conservative management should be continued, with regular (alternate day) monitoring of blood pressure, platelet count, serum creatinine and liver function tests, in addition to appropriate monitoring of the fetus. Possible indications for delivery include the following:

- Platelet: $<100 \times 10^9/l$
- Creatinine: >100 μmol/l
- ALT/AST: >50 iu/l
- Albumin: <20 g/l
- Symptoms, such as epigastric or right upper quadrant pain, or severe headache.
- Inability to control the blood pressure with maximal doses of three antihypertensive drugs.
- Fetal compromise.

In practice, there is no absolute cut-off point for the above blood test results that is applicable at all gestational ages. The closer to term the pregnancy, the less abnormal the result that could prompt delivery. In general, it is a balance between the risks of prematurity, a failed induction of labour and emergency Caesarean section, or an elective Caesarean section and the risks to the mother (developing a crisis related to pre-eclampsia such as HELLP syndrome, eclampsia, pulmonary oedema, renal impairment and placental abruption) and the fetus (placental abruption and intrauterine death) if the pregnancy is continued.

3.3 POSTPARTUM BREATHLESSNESS

You are asked to review a 36 year old Ghanaian woman on the postnatal ward. She had her fifth normal delivery 1 day previously and has complained to the midwives that she feels breathless. She had an uneventful pregnancy until 20 weeks' gestation when she required iron supplements for anaemia. At 36 weeks' gestation, her blood pressure was noted to be elevated (155/100 mmHg), having been normal at booking (135/85 mmHg). She was treated with methyldopa, 250 mg three times daily, which was stopped at delivery. She did not develop proteinuria and pre-eclampsia; bloods were persistently normal. She developed hypertension in the late third trimester of her last two pregnancies but has no significant past medical history of note. On closer questioning, she denies chest pain, has no cough and tells you the breathlessness has been getting gradually worse since delivery and that last night she was very breathless, except when she was breastfeeding her baby.

On examination, she is obese (her weight at booking was 120 kg) and apyrexial, with regular monitoring of blood pressure and alternate day platelet. Her jugular venous pressure (JVP) is not raised, there is no right ventricular heave, the apex is at the anterior axillary line and she has a gallup rhythm with a loud systolic murmur. There are bilateral fine crepitations at the bases of both lung fields. Mild ankle oedema is present, but no sacral oedema. Abdominal examination reveals a well-contracted uterus and no organomegaly.

1. What is the likely diagnosis?
2. What investigations would you request?
3. What would you expect these investigations to show?
4. Justify your subsequent management plan.

Answers

1. The breathlessness is most likely to be due to pulmonary oedema. The history is suggestive of orthopnoea (possibly relieved by sitting up to breastfeed). She is tachycardic and tachypnoeic, and has bibasal crackles, all of which support a diagnosis of pulmonary oedema. The differential diagnosis of postpartum pulmonary oedema includes peripartum cardiomyopathy, which is the most likely diagnosis. The risk factors in this case are obesity, multiparity and pregnancy-induced hypertension. The findings of an enlarged heart, systolic murmur (because of mitral and/or tricuspid regurgitation secondary to ventricular dilation) and gallup rhythm also support the diagnosis.

   There is long differential diagnosis for pulmonary oedema, including primary valvular causes, such as mitral regurgitation and mitral stenosis. The latter would cause a mid-diastolic murmur that might be overlooked in the presence of a tachycardia of 120 bpm. The other important cause to exclude is iatrogenic fluid overload. The differential diagnosis of breathlessness postpartum must include pulmonary embolism, but in the absence of chest pain and with the above clinical examination findings, this is unlikely.

2. Appropriate investigations would include the following:

   Electrocardiogram (ECG).
   Echocardiogram.
   Chest X-ray.
   Arterial blood gases.
   Full blood count (FBC).
   Urea and electrolytes.
   Serum creatinine.
   Liver function tests.

3. In peripartum cardiomyopathy, the echocardiographic features include the following:

   Global dilation of all four heart chambers.
   Left-ventricular dysfunction.
   The absence of any other cause of heart failure.

   The diagnostic criteria are as follows:

   Left-ventricular ejection fraction of <45%
   Fractional shortening of <30%
   Left-ventricular end diastolic pressure (LVEDP) of >2.7 cm/m^2

   The chest X-ray would show cardiomegaly and pulmonary oedema. The arterial blood gases might show hypoxia. It is important to repeat the "pre-eclampsia bloods" because pulmonary oedema could be a result of undiagnosed pre-eclampsia and hypoalbuminaemia, although the history does not suggest this. Cardiomyopathy with right heart involvement could cause deranged liver function tests because of "back pressure", but the transaminases are likely to be slightly abnormal after a normal delivery in any case. A FBC should be performed, especially because of her prior anaemia, grand multiparity and, therefore, her risk of postpartum haemorrhage, because unrecognised heavy bleeding at delivery could result in anaemia, which might exacerbate her dyspnoea and tachycardia.

4. She should be referred to a cardiologist. Initial management involves oxygen therapy, if hypoxic, and diuretics to treat the pulmonary oedema. Because she is postpartum, it is appropriate to start an angiotensin-converting enzyme (ACE) inhibitor. ACE inhibitors, although contraindicated in pregnancy, are safe to use in breastfeeding mothers. Treatment is started at a low dose and increased gradually if the blood pressure allows. Worsening heart failure and hypotension are indications for inotropes. Because one of the greatest risks in peripartum cardiomyopathy relates to thrombotic events, prophylactic heparin should be started immediately. Cardiac transplantation might be the only option in severe cases

that are unresponsive to conventional and full-supportive management. Most maternal deaths occur close to presentation. About 50% of patients have spontaneous and full recovery. The patient should be counselled about contraception and future pregnancy. The prognosis depends on whether there is normalization of the left-ventricular size and function within 6 months of delivery. Mortality is increased in those with persistent left-ventricular dysfunction. Women should be counselled against further pregnancy if the left-ventricle size and function do not return to normal, because there is a significant risk of recurrence (40–50%) and mortality (20%) [2]. The recurrence risk in women whose hearts return to normal size and function is lower (20%). However, the contractile reserve might be impaired, even if the left-ventricle size and function are normal. Subsequent pregnancies require high-risk collaborative care. Therefore, adequate effective contraception is important in all women until cardiology follow-up can differentiate the high-risk women from the moderate-risk women.

3.4 FETAL TACHYCARDIA

You are phoned by a midwife in a community clinic who is seeing a woman at 28 weeks gestation whose baby has a tachycardia of 180 bpm, measured using a hand-held sonicaid. The midwife tells you that the woman is taking tablets for a "thyroid problem".

1. What are the causes of fetal tachycardia?
2. How would decide whether this is fetal thyrotoxicosis?
3. How would you treat fetal thyrotoxicosis?

Answers

Fetal thyrotoxicosis is uncommon. The fetal risk is proportional to the level of maternal thyrotropin receptor-stimulating antibody. Beyond 20–24 weeks' gestation, the fetal thyroid can respond to this passively acquired antibody. Fetal thyrotoxicosis could present with intrauterine death premature delivery, craniosynostosis and impaired intellectual development or any of the features discussed below.

1. Fetal tachycardia should be confirmed on a CTG.

    Transient tachycardia might be due to fetal movements and appear as sustained accelerations on the CTG.

    True fetal tachycardia might be due to the following:
    • Infection.
    • Fetal distress/placental insufficiency.

- Administration of maternal drugs, such as beta-sympathomimetics.
- Fetal tachyarrythmia, especially supraventricular tachycardia, possibly associated with cardiac anomaly.
- Fetal thyrotoxicosis.

2. The features that suggest fetal thyrotoxicosis fall into two categories. First, the absence of other causes of tachycardia (e.g. no evidence of maternal infection or chorioamnionitis) and lack of relevant medication or a normal CTG apart from tachycardia, with no decelerations and normal variability and no other obvious cause for placental insufficiency, such as pre-eclampsia or abruptio placentae. Second, there might be specific features in the history or examination that point to fetal thyrotoxicosis, for example:

- Maternal thyrotoxicosis, either active or previously treated with radioactive iodine or surgery, such that there might still be circulating thyrotropin receptor-stimulating antibodies.
- Increased fetal movements, intrauterine growth restriction (IUGR) with oligohydramnios or goitre with polyhydramnios.
- Fetal hydrops points to longstanding tachycardia, but not specifically to fetal thyrotoxicosis.

The ultimate diagnosis of fetal hyperthyroidism is made by cordocentesis. This is only justified if there is sufficient clinical evidence to make the diagnosis likely, but insufficient evidence to make it certain, and prematurity precludes delivery. There are well-defined reference ranges for fetal thyroid function against which the results can be compared. Cordocentesis is more reliable than amniocentesis for assessing fetal thyroid status.

In this case, which is remote from term, treatment would be with carbimazole, orally administered to the mother: as it crosses the placenta it will suppress fetal thyroid activity. The dose is titrated against fetal tachycardia and movements. If the mother becomes clinically hypothyroid, she must also take thyroxine, which does not cross the placenta and so does not affect fetal thyroid function. Further cordocenteses can be considered, depending on the response to treatment and the gestational age. At delivery, cord thyroid function tests should be preformed, and a paediatric review initiated.

3. All women with active thyrotoxicosis or a history of Graves' disease that was treated by radioactive iodine or surgery should have TSH receptor-stimulating antibodies measured in early pregnancy. Those with a positive titre should be offered fetal monitoring after 24 weeks' gestation, perhaps in the form of maternal assessment of fetal movements, regular measurement of fetal heart rate and a growth scan in the third trimester. Cord

blood should be taken and a paediatric follow-up arranged, especially if the woman is taking antithyroid medication, which could have masked the effect of the antibodies *in utero*.

3.5 ABDOMINAL PAIN AND ANAEMIA

A 27 year old Nigerian woman attends the day assessment unit at 22 weeks' gestation complaining of abdominal pain. She has not booked, having returned from a 4 month stay in Nigeria 2 weeks previously. This is her third pregnancy; she had two uncomplicated pregnancies 1 year and 3 years ago, respectively, both within the UK, where she has been resident for 8 years. She tells you that she visited her local accident and emergency (A+E) department 3 days previously because of the abdominal pain and was told she had a urinary tract infection and prescribed amoxicillin (amoxycillin). The pain was no better, prompting her visit to the day assessment unit. While in Nigeria, she had felt tired and purchased some iron supplements. On examination, she is apyrexial and her heart rate is 76 bpm; the uterine size is consistent with the gestational age. She is tender in the right hypochondrium and has 1+ proteinuria. Her blood pressure is 128/76 mmHg. You review her results from the A+E department and notice that her Hb concentration was 9.2 g/dl and MCV was 86 fl. A urine culture was negative. You repeat the FBC: her Hb concentration is now 7.8 g/dl WBC and platelet count are normal. Biochemistry is normal apart from a bilirubin level of 54 μmol/l and a serum albumin level of 19 g/l. You organize an upper abdominal ultrasound, which reveals a normal liver, gall bladder and pancreas. There is mild hydronephrosis on the right, a normal kidney on the left and splenomegaly (16 cm).

1. Discuss the differential diagnosis and your management plan.

Answers

1. This woman has a normocytic anaemia and splenomegaly. The most likely diagnosis is malaria. Differential diagnoses include haemolytic anaemia, acute viral infection, portal hypertension and myeloproliferative disease. The raised bilirubin level suggests haemolysis; the falling Hb concentration suggests that this is acute. Investigation should include a peripheral blood smear to look for malarial parasites.

   Peripheral parasitaemia over 2% should be regarded as severe disease. Other investigations, if malaria is not confirmed, include a blood film, a Coombs' test for haemolytic anaemia and a reticulocyte count. Leukaemia is unlikely because of the normal WBC. Pre-eclampsia and HELLP syndrome are unlikely because of the normal blood pressure, normal platelet count and normal transaminases. Pre-eclampsia does not cause splenomegaly. A mild hydronephrosis is normal in pregnancy, but because of proteinuria, the midstream urine (MSU) should be repeated. Proteinuria occurs in malaria.

Plasmodium falciparum is responsible for the most severe disease in malaria. Immigrants from sub-Saharan Africa who have lived in the UK and return intermittently to Africa are likely to be nonimmune. Pregnant women, with little or no immunity, are at increased risk of developing severe disease compared with nonpregnant women. Maternal and perinatal mortality are increased. Pregnant women with malaria should be admitted for treatment because of their increased risk of hypoglycaemia and severe disease. Treatment depends on the Plasmodium type and the pattern of drug resistance in Nigerian malaria. Expert advice should be sought. Quinine is the drug of choice for *P. falciparum*. There is a particular risk of severe hypoglycaemia. Oral therapy is 10 mg/kg body weight three times daily for a minimum of 5 days, until clearance of parasitaemia. Intravenous therapy is 20 mg/kg body weight over 4 hours, followed by 10 mg/kg body weight over 4 hours three times daily.

If *P. falciparum* malaria is confirmed, management should include admission for treatment with intravenous quinine. The risks from severe disease in pregnancy include hypoglycaemia (particularly with intravenous quinine treatment), severe anaemia (this women's Hb concentration is falling fast), pulmonary oedema (the albumin level is already low), hyperpyrexia and cerebral malaria. In pregnancy, parasites sequester in the placenta, where infection might be very heavy. Malaria increases the risk of second-trimester miscarriage, premature labour and low birth weight. The Hb concentration and platelet count should be checked regularly. Blood glucose should be monitored initially and then every 2 hours when quinine is first commenced. ECG monitoring is advised during intravenous quinine administration because it could cause atrial fibrillation, conduction defects and heart block. A single treatment dose of pyrimethamine-sulfadoxine is given following parasite clearance. This patient should be counselled regarding the likely decline in her immunity to malaria because she is resident in the UK. If she wishes to return to an endemic area, such as Nigeria, she should take antimalarial prophylaxis in the same way as any UK resident.

3.6 ABNORMAL BLOOD GASES

Look at the arterial blood gas result performed at 28 weeks' gestation in a woman with dyspnoea, and answer the following questions:

pH: 7.38
HCO_3:   14 mmol/l
pCO_2:   2.7 kPa
pO_2:   14 kPa

1. Interpret the results.
2. Describe the changes that happen to pCO_2 in normal pregnancy.
3. Look at the results below and calculate the anion gap:

    Na: 139 mmol/l
    K: 4.5 mmol/l
    Cr: 120 μmol/l
    U: 8.7 mmol/l
    Cl: 107 mmol/l

4. In the light of the calculated anion gap, give three causes for the arterial blood gas (ABG) results.

Answers

1. This is a compensated metabolic acidosis: the pH is normal, but the bicarbonate concentration is low (normal range, 20–22 mmol/l), and the pCO_2 is low as a compensatory move to maintain neutrality.
2. The pCO_2 falls in normal pregnancy secondary to increased respiration. The nonpregnant normal range is usually 4.5–6 kPa; in pregnancy it is typically 3.5–4.5 kPa.
3. The anion gap defines the unmeasurable anions that maintain electro-neutrality. The calculation is as follows:

   $[Na + K] - [HCO_3 + Cl]$
   (i.e. 143.5 − 121 = 22.5)

   The normal anion gap is 6–12. Therefore, this acidosis is caused by an acid other than hydrochloric acid.
4. This is a compensated metabolic acidosis with a raised anion gap. Three causes to consider are as follows:

   a. Diabetic ketoacidosis – check the history for diabetes; test urine for ketones; measure blood sugar; and treat aggressively with intravenous rehydration using normal saline and intravenous insulin and potassium (to lower the glucose level and prevent hypokalaemia, because insulin carries potassium ions into cells).

b. Salicyclate poisoning – check the history for aspirin use or risk factors for deliberate overdose; and measure the salicyclate level.

c. Lactic acidosis – check the history and clinical examination findings for causes of and features of lactic acidosis (e.g. hypotension and septic shock; drugs, including metformin and antiretroviral agents, especially nucleoside reverse transcriptase inhibitors in highly active antiretroviral therapy (HAART)); and measure lactate levels; treat or remove the underlying cause.

3.7 ABDOMINAL PAIN AND ABNORMAL LIVER FUNCTION

A woman who is 37 weeks into her first pregnancy complains of feeling generally unwell for 3 days, with right upper quadrant pain. She has no other localizing symptoms and has never been ill before. On examination, she is afebrile and her pulse is 80 bpm and blood pressure is 140/90 mmHg; there is trace protein on urine dipstick analysis. These are her initial blood results:

ALT:	150 iu/l
AST:	120 iu/l
Bilirubin:	20 μmol/l
Albumin:	28 g/l
Creatinine:	78 μmol/l
Sodium:	138 mmol/l
Potassium:	4.2 mmol/l
Urea:	3.4 mmol/l
Urate:	0.68 mmol/l

1. List your first three differential diagnoses.
2. List the first three maternal investigations you would order, and briefly justify each.
3. You repeat the liver function tests 6 hours later. The results are shown below:

ALT:	786 iu/l
AST:	669 iu/l
Bilirubin:	27 μmol/l
Albumin:	27 g/l

What is your provisional diagnosis? Outline your immediate management.

ANSWERS

1. (a) HELLP syndrome.

(b) Acute fatty liver of pregnancy (AFLP).
(c) Viral hepatitis, e.g. hepatitis A.

2. (a) A FBC with film: a low platelet count would suggest PET or HELLP syndrome; intravascular haemolysis, as indicated by fragmented red blood cells on the film, would suggest HELLP syndrome; a raised WBC would suggest a infective cause, but a very high WBC supports AFLP.

(b) Clotting: abnormal clotting, especially prolonged INR would support incipient acute liver failure for which there are a large number of causes, but in this scenario AFLP must be strongly considered. Prothrombin is the clotting factor with the shortest half-life and, therefore, is the first to be affected when there is reduced liver manufacture. Abnormal clotting can also reflect DIC in association with HELLP syndrome.

(c) Glucose: hypoglycaemia can occur in AFLP because of the impaired ability of the failing liver to release glucose from glycogen breakdown or to make glucose form other sources, such as lactate and amino acids. Hypoglycaemia must not be overlooked, because otherwise it can cause impaired consciousness and even death.

3. The rapid deterioration in the liver function tests makes AFLP the most likely, and the most dangerous, diagnosis. Management is based on the following:

(a) Confirming the diagnosis.
(b) Delivering the baby.
(c) Managing the incipient liver failure.

At this point, if not already performed, blood should be taken for a viral hepatitis screen to include hepatitis A, B and C, cytomegalovirus, Epstein-Barr virus and human immunodeficiency virus (HIV). The renal function, glucose, clotting and FBC measurements should be repeated, and a group and save performed, in case delivery is required by Caesarean section or a bleeding diathesis ensues. The history should be checked carefully to ensure no medication, travel, contacts or past problems have been overlooked, and a thorough examination repeated, especially checking for signs of chronic liver disease.

AFLP affects 1 in 10,000 pregnancies and has a high case fatality ratio for both mother and baby. The best way to halt the disease process is to deliver the baby, which not only helps the maternal condition, but also removes the baby from a potentially hostile environment. Usually, delivery is initially attempted vaginally, and, pleasingly, induction of labour is often swift. If Caesarean section is necessary, for fetal or maternal reasons, the major issue of concern is the potential bleeding problems that can arise from performing major surgery in someone with incipient liver failure: whenever possible, a decision to perform Caesarean section should be made sooner rather than later, although in clinical practice this can be very difficult.

The paediatricians must be alerted to the likely maternal diagnosis of AFLP: in some cases, maternal AFLP is because of homozygosity of long-chain hydroxyacyl-Co A dehydrogenase deficiency (LCHAD) in the baby, the excess unmetabolised fetal fatty acids saturating the reduced (heterozygous) maternal enzyme level and resulting in acute liver failure; the baby needs investigation and a special diet devoid of long-chain fatty acids. Women in this situation have a 25% risk of recurrence of AFLP if they stay in the same partnership.

Women with AFLP can progress very rapidly to acute liver failure. They must be nursed very carefully, with hourly observations of all vital signs, careful observation for bleeding diathesis (e.g. bruising or bleeding, either spontaneously or from sites of minor trauma, such as venepuncture) and impaired conscious levels, capillary glucose measurements every 2 hours, and regular liver function tests with clotting measurements. Venous access should be secured with large-bore cannulae, and it is often sensible for a central line to be sited while clotting is still normal, to enable safe delivery of large quantities of 50% dextrose solution, which can be irritating to small peripheral veins. Usually, women should be managed on the delivery suite until the baby is born and then transferred to the most appropriate intensive care bed afterwards.

A multidisciplinary approach is important, including experienced obstetricians, anaesthetists, haematologists and hepatologists. If liver function continues to deteriorate, early contact with the regional liver transplant centre is vital: they are an invaluable source of advice on further investigation (e.g. whether other causes of liver failure, such as paracetamol overdose, Wilson's disease, alpha 1 antitrypsin deficiency, etc, must be considered) and management, and, if appropriate, can take over care as soon as delivery is expedited. They usually recommend an infusion of N-acetyl cysteine.

AFLP can be a frightening experience for the woman and her family, and so all efforts must be made to ensure that they are fully informed about what is happening. They will need follow-up, both to re-explain the events surrounding delivery and to consider future pregnancies.

3.8 DIABETES

A woman with longstanding diabetes attends your antenatal endocrine clinic. She is 12 weeks' pregnant. In her only other pregnancy, 7 years ago, she had a Caesarean section at 30 weeks' gestation for severe pre-eclampsia; her son weighed 1.4 kg and is now well after a stormy course in the neonatal intensive care unit (NICU). She has background retinopathy, renal impairment (nonpregnant creatinine level, 170 μmol/l) and hypertension. She has excellent diabetic control, with a glycosylated haemoglobin (HbA_{1c}) at the upper limit of normal; she takes enalapril for hypertension.

1. What baseline tests do you do today; give one rationale for each test?
2. What is her risk of the following:
   (a) Renal deterioration
   (b) Developing pre-eclampsia
   (c) Delivering preterm
3. List three ways you might be able to distinguish pre-eclampsia from a deterioration in renal function.

Answers

1. The following baseline tests today should be done today:
   (a) Blood pressure measurement – uncontrolled hypertension is a predictor of poor pregnancy outcome, with increased risk of renal deterioration, IUGR and prematurity.
   (b) Antiphospholipid screening – although diabetic renal disease is a strong risk factor for recurrent severe, early onset pre-eclampsia, this does not preclude other important causes.
   (c) Fetal ultrasound scan – accurate assessment of gestational age is vital, especially as there is a substantial risk of premature delivery. In addition, an early check for major anomalies is important.
   (d) Baseline assessment of renal function – to give accurate advice regarding outcome of the pregnancy, and as a baseline value.
   (e) Baseline measurements of platelet count and liver function – against which to compare subsequent results if pre-eclampsia supervenes.
   (f) Dilated fundoscopy – if the retinopathy has progressed and there is now proliferative retinopathy, this needs active treatment to protect visual acuity.
   (g) Urine analysis for proteinuria and protein to creatinine ratio – to characterise renal involvement and acts as a baseline level if it progresses later in the pregnancy.

2. Advice regarding risks is based on the fact that she has moderate renal impairment (i.e. a serum creatinine level between 125 μmol/l and 250 μmol/l) and hypertension, with previous early onset pre-eclampsia.

The risks will be approximately as follows:

(a) Renal deterioration: 25%
(b) Pre-eclampsia: 50%
(c) Preterm delivery: 50%

3. The following help to distinguish pre-eclampsia from renal deterioration:

Falling platelet count in pre-eclampsia.
Abnormal liver function tests in pre-eclampsia.
Rising uric acid level.

Worsening hypertension, increasing proteinuria, deteriorating renal function and placental insufficiency (IUGR and oligohydramnios) occur in both diabetic renal disease and pre-eclampsia and cannot be used to distinguish the two conditions.

3.9 FACIAL WEAKNESS

A pregnant woman presents with recent, sudden-onset, unilateral facial weakness.

1. What is the differential diagnosis?
2. What aspects of the history and examination help to establish which of your differential diagnoses are correct?
3. Discuss the symptoms and signs that might be associated with the most common cause of facial weakness in pregnancy?
4. Outline the treatment options.

Answers

1. This is a VIIth nerve palsy. The differential diagnosis is either an upper motor neurone lesion (UML) or a lower motor neurone lesion (LML).
2. In a UML, frontalis and obicularis oris are spared, so that she will be able to close her eye and furrow her brow. A UML is rarely isolated, so the history and examination will usually localize other neurological deficits, especially in the long tracts or other cranial nerves. A LML causes weakness of all the muscles of the face, so that eye closure, including blinking, and furrowing of the brow are lost.
3. Bell's palsy is the commonest cause of facial weakness in pregnancy. Outside pregnancy there are 2 in 10,000 cases per year, but it is more common in pregnancy, presumably because of compression associated with oedema as the nerve passes through the narrow,

bony canal of the mastoid process. The following are common and should be sought:

- Pain in or behind the ear, with or without the typical rash of herpes zoster.
- Numbness on the affected side of the face.
- Loss of taste on ipsilateral anterior two-thirds of the tongue.
- Hyperacusis.

Less commonly, Bell's palsy can be associated with sarcoidosis, Lyme disease, demyelination or space-occupying lesions.

4. Treatment should include the following:

   (a) Protection of the cornea from particles in the air (because of the loss of the blink reflex) and from damage by bedclothing while sleeping: an eye patch is advised until the eye recovers.
   (b) Use of articial tears for corneal dryness.
   (c) Prednisolone improves the proportion of people making a good recovery from 80% to 97%, by reducing the oedema. Ideally, it is started within 72 hours of onset, although some improvement has been recorded if the drug is started up to 7 days after onset. The dose is usually 1 mg/kg body weight, with a maximum dose of 80 mg, for 1 week, and then it is tapered and stopped during the next 7 days.
   (d) Even if there is no clinical evidence of herpes infection, aciclovir should be started, 800 mg five times daily for 5 days, as herpes is thought to be a common aetiological factor in Bell's plasy.

It is important to explain that this is not a stroke and reassure the patient that there is a good chance of full recovery.

The following are useful websites:

http://www.bellspalsy.org.uk website accessed 17/10/06: UK-based website of the Bell's Palsy association, with useful information for sufferers of Bell's Palsy.

REFERENCES

1. RCOG Green top Guideline no 10A Management of severe pre-eclampsia/eclampsia March 2006.
2. Elkayam U, Tummala P, Rao K. Maternal and fetal outcomes of subsequent pregnancies in women with peripartum cardiomyopathy. *New Engl J Med* 2001; **344:** 1567–71.

Chapter 4
Essay Questions

4.1 MITRAL VALVE REPLACEMENT

Discuss the management of a 23 year old primiparous woman with a metal Starr-Edwards mitral valve replacement who is receiving maintenance therapy with warfarin and who presents at 5 weeks' gestation.

Model Answer

The optimal management of women with metal heart-valve replacements in pregnancy is controversial because the interests of the mother and the fetus are in conflict. These women require life-long anticoagulation and this must be continued in pregnancy because of the increased risk of thrombosis. Thrombosis could involve the valve itself or lead to embolic phenomena, including transient ischaemic attacks and cerebrovascular accidents. Warfarin crosses the placenta and is associated with warfarin embryopathy if given between 6 weeks' and 12 weeks' gestation. The risk of teratogenesis is about 5%. Warfarin is also associated with an increased risk of miscarriage, still-birth and fetal intracerebral haemorrhage. There is some evidence that the adverse fetal effects of warfarin are related to the dose required to maintain the maternal INR over 2, with doses of warfarin in excess of 5mg associated with higher risks of teratogenesis, miscarriage and stillbirth. Heparin, whether unfractionated heparin (UH) or low-molecular-weight heparin (LMWH), is associated with increased risks of valve thrombosis and embolic events, even in full anticoagulant doses, compared with warfarin. However, because it does not cross the placenta, there are no adverse effects on the fetus. The risk of valve thrombosis and embolic events is also related to both the site and the type of valve prosthesis. Thus, valves in the mitral position are associated with a higher risk than those in the aortic position. Also, the newer bi-leaflet valves (e.g. Carbomedics) have a lower thrombotic risk than older, first-generation ball-and-cage valves (e.g. Starr-Edwards) or Bjork-Shiley valves. Other issues that must be considered are the risk of premature labour and the possibility of urgent delivery in a mother who is fully warfarinized.

The safest option for this mother is to continue warfarin throughout pregnancy. This is because she has a thrombogenic valve in the mitral position. The control of the warfarin therapy should be extremely tight, avoiding periods of undercoagulation or overcoagulation and maintaining the INR between 2.0 and 3.5. This will necessitate very regular visits to an anticoagulation clinic. Other management strategies include replacing warfarin with high-dose subcutaneous or intravenous UH or a subcutaneous LMWH, either from 6–12 weeks' gestation to avoid warfarin embryopathy or throughout the pregnancy. Full-dose intravenous UH is obviously not practical for prolonged periods, but some pregnancies in women with metal valves can be managed on full anticoagulant doses of LMWH (e.g. enoxaparin, 1 mg/kg body weight/twice daily).

Whichever management option is chosen, warfarin should be discontinued and substituted with heparin 10 days before delivery to enable clearance of warfarin from the fetal circulation. For delivery itself, heparin therapy is decreased or interrupted. Warfarin is recommenced 2–3 days postpartum. Heparin can be discontinued once the INR reaches 2.0 or greater. In the event of bleeding or the need for urgent delivery in a fully anticoagulated patient, warfarin can be reversed with fresh frozen plasma (FFP) and vitamin K, and heparin with protamine sulphate. However, vitamin K should be avoided if possible because it renders the woman extremely difficult to anticoagulate with warfarin after delivery. Women with metal valve replacements all require prophylaxis of endocarditis with antibiotics during delivery, regardless of the mode of delivery.

When this woman presents at 5 weeks' gestation, she should be fully counselled about the risks and benefits of the various therapeutic options to both her and her baby. If, despite directive counselling advising her to continue warfarin throughout pregnancy, she prefers to replace warfarin with a LMWH, this should be achieved before 6 weeks' gestation if possible. She should be taught how to self-administer the heparin injections. Low-dose aspirin (75 mg/day) could be added as an extra antithrombotic agent. She should be advised of the potential risks of all strategies, and if she elects to continue with warfarin, serial ultrasound scans should be offered because of the risk of warfarin embryopathy and intracerebral haemorrhage in the baby. She should be advised to attend hospital immediately if she goes into labour or develops any new symptoms. If the underlying need for her mitral valve replacement relates to congenital heart disease, she should be offered fetal cardiology scanning to exclude congenital heart disease in the fetus. Postpartum, she should be reassured that breastfeeding is safe with both heparin and warfarin therapy. Future contraception should be discussed.

4.2 SICKLE CELL DISEASE

Describe your counselling and antenatal management plan for a 32 year old primiparous women with sickle cell disease who is 12 weeks' pregnant.

Model Answer

Sickle cell disease is a genetic haemolytic anaemia. There are several forms of sickle cell disease, of which the most common are sickle cell anaemia (SS), haemoglobin SC disease and sickle beta-thalassaemia (S thal) disease. Women with sickle cell disease have an increased risk of morbidity, both maternal and perinatal, and mortality in pregnancy. These risks relate to an increased predisposition to both pre-eclampsia and growth restriction. There is also an increased risk of sickle cell crises in pregnancy, which most commonly cause bone pain. Sickle cell crises can be precipitated by infection, dehydration, hypoxia, cold and acidosis.

Management should occur in a joint clinic, or in conjunction, with a haematologist who has expertise in the management of sickle cell pregnancies and begins with a detailed past medical history. Women with SS have a chronic haemolytic anaemia, but most are generally healthy between episodes of crisis, the frequency of which is enormously variable. However, some women have retinopathy, leg ulcers, renal involvement and previous strokes. Having established the woman's baseline health status, explain the increased risk of crises in pregnancy and the need for her to present to hospital to have these aggressively managed. Reassure her regarding the safety of opiate analgesia in pregnancy if it is required to treat sickle cell crises. She should also be advised to avoid well-known precipitants (cold and dehydration) and attend hospital to have any intercurrent infection treated rapidly. She should be offered echocardiography, because asymptomatic pulmonary hypertension (PHT) occurs in up to 30% of people with sickle cell disease: PHT has a 30–50% mortality rate in the puerperium.

The genetics of sickle cell disease should be explained and electrophoresis recommended for her partner, to ascertain the risk of her carrying a fetus with SS, SC disease or S thal disease. If she has

SS and her partner has a sickle cell trait, the risk of her fetus having SS is 50%. Prenatal diagnosis with chorionic villus sampling (CVS) or amniocentesis can be offered.

The obstetric risks of miscarriage, uteroplacental insufficiency and pre-eclampsia should be explained, in addition to the need for regular antenatal visits and serial ultrasound scans of the fetus to monitor growth. Many women with SS are offered elective delivery at 38 weeks' gestation to avoid the (small) risk of late intrauterine death. Therefore, and because of the increased risk of pre-eclampsia and IUGR, the rate of Caesarean section is increased. Women with SS and SC disease are also at increased risk of thromboembolic events and should receive prophylactic LMWH after a Caesarean section, if admitted with a sickle cell crisis or for any other reason. She should have an antenatal appointment with an obstetric anaesthetist to discuss the benefits of regional analgesia for both vaginal delivery and Caesarean section. In labour, she should have good analgesia and be well hydrated, usually with intravenous fluids.

All women with sickle cell disease should receive folic acid (5 mg) throughout pregnancy because they have a haemolytic anaemia and therefore their folate requirements are high. Because they have undergone "autosplenectomy", they also require prophylactic penicillin, which should be continued or started in pregnancy.

The role of exchange transfusion for SS in pregnancy is very controversial. There is some evidence that routine exchange transfusion reduces the risk of sickle cell crises, by reducing the percentage of Haemoglobin S. However, the risk of transfusion reactions in those who have received multiple transfusions is high and some say prohibitive. Other strategies include the use of "top-up" transfusions for severe anaemia only.

If a crisis does occur in pregnancy, it should be managed in hospital with intravenous fluids and analgesia. A rigorous search for, and treatment of, underlying infective precipitants is indicated. When a crisis presents with chest pain, this could represent infection, infarction or pain related to "sickling" alone, or more commonly a combination of all three factors.

In summary, this is a high-risk pregnancy and thus advice to the patient and antenatal care should reflect the need for increased surveillance of both mother and fetus.

4.3 HYPERTHYROIDISM

You are asked to review a 29 year old nurse in the first trimester of pregnancy, whose blood tests suggest hyperthyroidism. Discuss the clinical differential diagnosis, prognosis and management options; explain your rationale.

Model Answer

In broad terms, the differential diagnosis includes deterioration or relapse of previously diagnosed thyroid disease, newly diagnosed autoimmune thyrotoxicosis, gestational or biochemical thyrotoxicosis related to hyperemesis gravidarum, molar pregnancy and other rarer causes of thyrotoxicosis, including thyroiditis, malignancy, solitary active nodule and fictitious thyrotoxicosis.

A detailed history and examination should help in reaching the correct diagnosis. If she has previously had Graves' disease, she could be experiencing a relapse. Relapse is not infrequent in the first trimester, and is thought to reflect the altered maternal immune state: clinical disease activity follows the titre of thyrotropin receptor- stimulating antibodies, which increases in the first trimester. If she is currently taking antithyroid medication, relapse could also be because of impaired absorption secondary to pregnancy-associated vomiting or inappropriate cessation of tablets (commonly on the basis of unfounded concern about teratogenesis). A completely new diagnosis of autoimmune thyrotoxicosis is uncommon in early pregnancy, because untreated disease is associated with reduced libido and fertility. The presence of vomiting and associated symptoms points to hyperemesis gravidarum (HG), which is the commonest cause of hyperthyroidism in the first trimester in women who do not give a prepregnancy history of thyroid disease; rarely, nausea and vomiting are a dominant feature in autoimmune thyroid disease, and care should be taken to distinguish the two conditions.

The clinical symptoms and signs of thyrotoxicosis and pregnancy can be similar, and should be interpreted carefully. Weight loss despite a good diet, failure of tachycardia to settle with Valsalva manoeuvre and onycholysis are helpful indicators of active hyperthyroidism. Eye signs and pretibial myxoedema do not reflect the activity of Graves' disease. Other symptoms and signs of thyrotoxicosis are not useful clinical discriminators between pregnancy and hyperthyroidism: fatigue, anxiety, emotional lability, heat intolerance, sweating, warm extremities and amenorrhoea are common in both. Vomiting is occasionally a feature of hyperthyroidism, so care must be taken to separate it from the more common HG. The presence of a small goitre is common in pregnancy. But, a large goitre or a palpable thyroid nodule could point to the diagnoses of multinodular goitre, toxic nodular adenoma or even thyroid malignancy. In this case, a thyroid ultrasound might be helpful: cystic lesions in association with hyperthyroidism make malignancy unlikely. However, if there are solid nodules, fine-needle aspiration (FNA) can, and indeed should, be safely employed during pregnancy to exclude malignancy. Radioactive iodine-uptake tests are contraindicated in pregnancy (as discussed later). If the FNA result is benign, she requires treatment with antithyroid medication in the usual way (see below). If the FNA result is malignant, she should be offered surgery. If, however, the report is "cellular", the management choices are more difficult because it could still be a malignant nodule: high-dose thyroxine, to suppress tumour growth, should not be employed in this woman because she has clinical hyperthyroidism.

The presence of thyroid autoantibodies supports a diagnosis of autoimmune hyperthyroidism, but is not sufficiently specific to confirm it. Similarly, a family history of thyroid disease supports this as a possible diagnosis.

The prognosis of the hyperthyroidism depends on its cause and how quickly thyroid dysfunction can be controlled. A number of observational studies in women with autoimmune thyrotoxicosis suggest that if hyperthyroidism remains poorly controlled, both maternal and fetal complications, such as thyroid storm, congestive cardiac failure, hypertensive disease of pregnancy, premature labour, small for gestational age infants and stillbirth, seem to be increased. The outcome is worse in pregnancies in which thyroid disease is never controlled, compared with those in which euthyroidism is achieved, but both of these patient groups have poorer outcomes than pregnancies in which thyroid disease is controlled before conception [1]. Although these studies might be flawed with confounding variables, and lack appropriate control subjects, it seems sensible to achieve control as soon as possible. If this nurse has a relapse or new diagnosis of hyperthyroidism, she should take either carbimazole or propylthiouracil (PTU). Recent evidence shows that these drugs are equally effective in pregnancy, without evidence of teratogenicity or fetal hypothyroidism, unless large doses are used: older literature, which imply there are risks of aplasia cutis and high placental transfer with PTU, but not carbimazole, are now discredited [2,3]. Indeed, depending on how early in the first trimester this woman is, use of antithyroid medication might reduce her risk of teratogenesis compared with women who do not become euthyroid during the first trimester [4]. Thyroid surgery can be performed in pregnancy, although it is usually reserved for women who have a symptomatic goitre, malignant disease or failed medical treatment. Radioactive iodine is absolutely contraindicated in this woman: iodine crosses the placenta and is actively taken up by the fetal thyroid once it begins functioning at around 8–10 weeks' gestation; radioactive iodine irreversibly destroys the fetal thyroid, with devastating consequences.

Biochemical hyperthyroidism is common in HG and has a good prognosis. In approximately 40% of women with HG, there is a raised free thyroxine (fT_4) level and/or suppressed thyroid-stimulating hormone (TSH) level, sometimes with a very high fT_4 level (80 pmol/l). The usual clinical picture of a woman with hyperemesis is someone who is listless, tired and washed out, which is not a common scenario in other forms of thyrotoxicosis. There are no goitre, tremor or eye signs; if present, tachycardia is secondary to dehydration, weight loss is secondary to poor nutritional intake and warm peripheries is secondary to the vasodilatation of pregnancy; the symptoms are clearly of recent onset and do not antedate the pregnancy. If there is clinical doubt concerning the differential diagnosis of thyroid dysfunction, the absence of thyroid antiperoxidase, antithyroglobulin autoantibodies and TSH receptor antibodies supports the diagnosis of hyperemesis.

Treatment of hyperemesis is centred on correcting the metabolic insults of prolonged vomiting and preventing further vomiting. There is no place for the use of antithyroid medication in hyperemesis: the thyroid abnormality is not usually long lasting. If antithyroid drugs are used for the treatment of human chorionic gonadotrophin (HCG)-induced hyperthyroidism [5], they are either ineffective or required in extremely high doses to achieve biochemical euthyroidism [6] (which might result in sufficient transplacental passage to cause fetal hypothyroidism). Thyroid function tests must be monitored serially, to ensure that they resolve as hyperemesis settles: clearly, if they do not, alternative explanations for the abnormality must be sought [7].

As part of the investigations of this nurse, a pelvic ultrasound examination is invaluable. Both multiple pregnancy and molar pregnancy are more likely to be associated with hyperemesis and hyperthyroidism. Details of her history, including ethnicity, past obstetric history, assisted conception and family history, could point to increased risk of either of these events. In the case of a molar pregnancy, the general prognosis clearly depends on the histological assessment, but is likely to be good, even if she has choriocarcinoma because it is usually highly responsive to methotrexate-based chemotherapy. The first line of management involves surgical evacuation of the uterus. Depending on the severity of the symptoms of hyperthyroidism, she might also need supportive measures, such as rehydration, antipyretics and beta-blockade. Usually, the symptoms will regress following surgery.

If the clinical picture is unusual, especially if there is a poor response to treatment, the possibility of Munchausen's disease, with self-administration of large amounts of thyroxine tablets should be considered. This is a difficult diagnosis to establish, and should be approached sensitively.

In summary, the most likely differential diagnosis is autoimmune thyroid disease or HG, although other less common causes of hyperthyroidism must be considered. Management should be based on a careful history and examination, probably involving an endocrinologist, or a physician or obstetrician with an interest in the medical problems of pregnancy.

4.4 DIABETES

Explain the points that should be discussed during prepregnancy counselling of women with diabetes. Which of these do you consider to be the most important, and why? How can you encourage women to adopt these measures?

Model Answer

The principles of diabetic management in pregnancy relate to the effect of the pregnancy on the diabetes and the effect of the diabetes on the mother and baby.

Pregnancy affects diabetes by increasing the insulin requirement, accelerating diabetic eye and renal diseases (usually temporarily, unless microvascular disease is already advanced), exacerbating hypertension, increasing the incidence of hypoglycaemia and lowering the threshold at which diabetic ketoacidosis occurs.

Diabetes affects the pregnancy by increasing the likelihood of miscarriage, major structural anomaly, pre-eclampsia, prematurity, birth trauma, Caesarean section, admission to neonatal intensive care and the so-called "minor problems" of pregnancy, such as thrush, heartburn, peripheral oedema, carpal tunnel syndrome and urinary tract infection [8].

Many of these problems can be minimized by achieving exemplary diabetic glycaemic control before conception and maintaining this throughout pregnancy. This is the most important principle in the management of diabetic pregnancy. If diabetic control is good at conception, with premeal values less than ~6 mmol/l, 2-hour postmeal levels less than ~8 mmol/l and glycosylated haemoglobin (HbA_{1c}) within the normal range, the outcome for the pregnancy in relation to miscarriage and structural anomaly is comparable with the general population, which is 20% and 3%, respectively. However, if a pregnancy is not planned, and conception occurs when control is less tight than this, the frequency of these outcomes increases approximately in relation to the level of control; for example, if HbA_{1c} is over 10%, the risks are around 75% and 30–50%, respectively. The cornerstone of management in diabetic pregnancy is, therefore, preconceptual planning. Target glucose measurements must be set, and the patient assisted in attaining them by optimizing her diet, exercising regularly and adjusting her treatment. Women on oral hypoglycaemic agents might need to add in, or switch to, insulin. Blood pressure should also be brought under tight control before conception, either using agents that are safe in pregnancy or by advising the woman to stop them as soon as a pregnancy test is positive. If she is taking cholesterol-lowering agents, she must be advised to stop these before pregnancy. Low-dose aspirin, for prophylaxis against pre-eclampsia, should be discussed so that the woman knows the rationale and when to commence it. General health issues pertinent to pregnancy must be discussed, including smoking, alcohol intake, rubella immunity, haemoglobinopathy screening, risks of aneuploidy and high-dose folate supplementation. Women should be given a contact point for accessing the antenatal endocrine services as soon as they are pregnant.

One of the major challenges in the care of young women with diabetes is to know how best to deliver this information to them, in a format that is acceptable and achievable. There are likely to be many different solutions, depending on local populations, but in most cases, preconceptual clinics must be promoted by a broad multidisciplinary team in a variety of settings and, possibly, in different local languages. This could include any health professional who comes into contact with women with diabetes, such as adult and adolescent endocrinology services, obstetric professionals, primary care teams, pharmacists and social services. Fundamental to the success of preconceptual care is contraception, which should be reliable and acceptable, in addition to quickly reversible when discontinued and safe in relation to diabetes.

4.5 POLYURIA AND POLYDYPSIA

A 34 year old primiparous women presents to the day assessment unit at 36 weeks' gestation complaining of excessive thirst and polyuria. You take a thorough history and establish that she is drinking up to 10 l of water daily. She is also passing vast quantities of urine and says that she wakes every 1 hour at night to pass urine.

Explain your differential diagnosis and outline what investigations you would perform.

Model Answer

The differential diagnosis of polyuria includes diuretic therapy, hyperglycaemia (diabetes mellitus), hypercalcaemia, hypokalaemia and diabetes insipidus (DI). In the absence of hyperglycaemia, the most likely diagnosis is DI. The incidence DI in pregnancy is approximately the same as in the nonpregnant female population (i.e. 1 in 15,000).

DI is caused by a relative deficiency of vasopressin (antidiuretic hormone [ADH]). There are four types, as follows:

Central – (cranial) due to deficient production of ADH from the posterior pituitary.

Nephrogenic – due to ADH resistance and most commonly associated with chronic renal disease.

Transient – due to increased vasopressinase production by the placenta or decreased vasopressinase breakdown by the liver. This form of DI is found in association with pre-eclampsia and HELLP syndrome or acute fatty liver of pregnancy (AFLP), and regresses after delivery.

Psychogenic – resulting from compulsive drinking of water and consequent polyuria.

Pregnancy could unmask previously subclinical DI. In those with established DI, there is a tendency to deterioration during pregnancy. The most likely diagnosis in this case is either unmasking of previous subclinical cranial DI, transient DI related to pregnancy or compulsive drinking of water.

The patient should be admitted to confirm and document the extent of polyuria and polydypsia. Urea, electrolytes, serum glucose and calcium should be checked. Paired samples of plasma and urine should be sent for estimation of osmolality.

The fundamental problem in DI is failure to concentrate the urine (because of deficient ADH). Confirmation of a diagnosis of DI is straightforward if the plasma osmolality (>295 mOsm/kg) or serum sodium (>145 mmol/l) is inappropriately raised in the presence of polyuria and a low urine osmolality (<300 mOsm/kg). This excludes compulsive drinking of water. However, often the plasma osmolality is normal (remembering that in pregnancy the upper limit of normal falls from about 285 mOsm/kg to 275 mOsm/kg). If fluid intake can be restricted so that plasma osmolality increases, an inability to concentrate the urine confirms a diagnosis of DI. In nonpregnant women, diagnosis is conventionally with a fluid-deprivation test, in which the patient is not allowed to drink for 15–22 hours, during which time serial weights, urine and plasma osmolalities are measured. Following dehydration and a loss of 3–5% of body weight, ADH is stimulated and urine concentration occurs in those without DI and in those with psychogenic DI. In pregnancy, such dehydration is potentially hazardous and a "short" water deprivation test (e.g. overnight) might be all that is required to demonstrate an increasing urine osmolality (>700 mOsmol/kg should be considered normal) with normal plasma osmolality, and thus exclude cranial and nephrogenic DI.

To differentiate between cranial and nephrogenic DI, administration of a synthetic analogue of vasopressin desmopressin (10–20 μg intranasally) is used. This will result in concentration of urine in cranial DI, and to a greater extent in patients without DI, but not in those with nephrogenic DI (who remain polyuric). Desmopressin use is safe for diagnosis or treatment of DI in pregnancy.

A confirmed or suspected diagnosis of new-onset DI in pregnancy should prompt a search for pre-eclampsia and AFLP, in particular.

4.6 SYSTEMIC LUPUS ERYTHEMATOSUS

A woman with systemic lupus erythematosus (SLE) comes to see you for prepregnancy advice. She is taking prednisolone (5 mg/day), ranitidine (300 mg/day) for reflux oesophagitis and codydramol for pain. She is otherwise well. She has never been pregnant.

What advice would you give her?

Model Answer

Advice to a woman with SLE would relate to the effect of the autoimmune condition on her pregnancy, both from her and from her baby's perspective, the effect of being pregnant on the SLE and the safety of medication during pregnancy and lactation. It is also important to cover general issues, including rubella immunity, haemoglobinopathy status, folate supplementation and smoking cessation.

Establish how the SLE has affected her, in particular whether there is renal involvement or hypertension, thrombocytopenia or other haematological problems, neurological problems (especially psychosis), a history of previous thromboembolic episodes and her autoantibody profile. Women with SLE have an increased risk of pre-eclampsia, the magnitude of the risk being determined by the extent of renal involvement and hypertension. Additional monitoring of blood pressure, proteinuria and fetal growth, including uterine artery waveform assessment should be advised. There is also a place for advising low-dose aspirin (75 mg daily), which in a recent meta-analysis was shown to reduce perinatal mortality, in addition to the incidence of pre-eclampsia. If she has had a major flare of SLE recently, especially a renal flare, she should be advised to delay pregnancy for 6 months.

The most important antibodies to consider are those related to the antiphospholipid syndrome, anticardiolipin and lupus anticoagulant, and anti-Ro and anti-La. If she has positive antiphospholipid antibodies on two occasions at least 6 weeks apart, she has an increased risk of first and second trimester miscarriage, intrauterine growth restriction, pre-eclampsia and later pregnancy loss. In women who have had recurrent first trimester loss in association with antiphospholipid antibodies, the correct management would be low-dose aspirin plus a thromboprophylactic dose of a LMWH. In this woman who has not had any obstetric disasters (or successes), the role of heparin is less certain, and the decision should therefore be based on joint discussion with the woman. Heparin-induced thrombocytopenia is extremely rare with LMWH, as is the risk of symptomatic vertebral collapse because of heparin-associated osteopenia (0.04%). Because she is taking prednisolone, she could already be at risk of osteoporosis, and it might be worth performing a prepregnancy baseline bone densitometry scan before deciding on the use of heparin.

Anti-Ro and anti-La antibodies have a 2% risk of causing congenital heart block and a 5% risk of causing neonatal cutaneous lupus. Once one pregnancy has been affected, the risk in a subsequent pregnancy rises to 20%. The fetal heart rate should be monitored from 14 weeks' gestation: heart block is not thought to occur before then, because the conducting system is not sufficiently developed. Preferably, monitoring should allow assessment of the atrial and ventricular rates, using M-mode Doppler imaging, which is present on most modern ultrasound machines used in antenatal departments. If there is a discrepancy between the atrial and the ventricular rates, or a fetal bradycardia is detected, referral should be made to a specialist unit. Intrauterine treatment is rarely successful, and early delivery could be indicated. In severe cases, hydrops fetalis might develop.

Autoimmune conditions can flare in the first trimester and postpartum, and are often relatively quiescent during the rest of the pregnancy. Women should conceive when they are in remission, and not within 6 months of a renal flare. SLE could deteriorate in the second half of pregnancy, and this can sometimes present confusion with pre-eclampsia if hypertension and proteinuria are worsening. In the postnatal period, women should accept all constructive help at home and be prepared to adjust their medication if a flare occurs. Flares can be especially distressing at this time if they involve the hands so that handling the baby is difficult.

The weight gain of pregnancy might make weight-bearing joints more painful, although in some women this is counterbalanced by an increased range of movement, presumably because of hormonally driven relaxation or softening of tissues surrounding them.

Prednisolone is safe in pregnancy, and the woman must be advised to continue it. Placental metabolism ensures that very little reaches the fetus, especially at this low dose [5 mg daily]. There are reassuring data about the lack of teratogenesis: reports suggesting that steroid do cause teratogenesis were confounded by the underlying conditions requiring treatment, the use of unconventional steroids and very diverse, and apparently unrelated, congenital abnormalities. There are a number of important maternal issues regarding prednisolone use in pregnancy, as follows:

- Steroid-induced hypertension could be confused with pre-eclampsia; blood pressure should be monitored more closely than normal.
- Steroid-induced glycaemia increases the risk of gestational diabetes. There should be a lower threshold for looking for diabetes.
- Adrenal suppression means that additional steroids should be given to cover stressful events, such as labour and delivery, significant antepartum haemorrhage, etc. This is usually hydrocortisone, 50 mg intravenously four times daily from the onset of the "stress" until 24 hours after the event is complete.
- Steroids and pregnancy each increase the risk of varicella pneumonitis if chickenpox develops. Women taking steroids who do not know if they have had chickenpox should have their immunity checked. If they are susceptible, they should avoid cases of chickenpox and immediately seek advice regarding the use of varicella zoster immunoglobulin (VZIG) and/or aciclovir if exposure occurs.

Ranitidine is safe in all trimesters of pregnancy and should be continued. Indigestion in pregnancy might exacerbate any pre-existing symptoms and make interpretation of steroid-induced gastritis difficult.

Codydramol is safe to continue. Constipation in pregnancy might be worsened by the codeine component. Women should be warned of this, and might consider a trial of paracetamol alone. She must be warned against using a nonsteroidal anti-inflammatory drug (NSAID) as an alternative, because it could cause fetal renal artery vasoconstriction or premature closure of the patent ductus arteriosus (PDA).

Give her general prepregnancy advice, including folate supplementation, smoking cessation and reducing alcohol intake in pregnancy. Offer screening for thalassaemia and sickle cell disease, rubella and diabetes, and take baseline measurements of renal and liver function and a full blood count. Depending on her age, issues regarding trisomy 21 should be discussed. Ensure that a letter summarizing all the issues discussed is sent to the patient and copied to the other teams involved in her care, including the rheumatologists and the general practitioner (GP). Give her a contact telephone number and the opportunity to return if further queries arise or as soon as she conceives.

4.7 DEEP VENOUS THROMBOSIS

You are asked to make a management plan for a woman who is 38 weeks' pregnant and has just been diagnosed with a large iliofemoral deep vein thrombosis (DVT). Discuss your options and any difficulties you perceive.

Model Answer

Management of acute DVT at term can be challenging, because labour and delivery increase the risk of further thrombosis, but anticoagulation can restrict analgesia and increase the risk of haemorrhage and haematoma.

This patient must be fully assessed. Risk factors for thrombosis must be reviewed (e.g. age, obesity, concurrent medical problems, family and personal histories, immobility, etc) and minimized where possible (e.g. maintaining mobility, treating infection and stopping smoking). The obstetric history must also be reviewed, and any further obstetric problems that might influence delivery should be identified; the likelihood of a vaginal delivery should be assessed. Any previous partograms should be reviewed. Ideally, a Caesarean section should be avoided because this increases the risk of thrombosis through the attendant pelvic vein trauma, immobility, dehydration and infection. However, an emergency Caesarean increases these risks more than an elective Caesarean, the latter also has a potential advantage over the former because there can be a minimal delay in administration of anticoagulation.

A thrombophilia screen should be carried out, preferably before the initiation of anticoagulation. Although this might be difficult to interpret accurately in pregnancy and in the presence of a thrombus, it is important to attempt to identify high-risk thrombophilic states, such as antithrombin deficiency, homozygosity for factor V Leiden and multiple heterozygous states: a family history of thrombosis or identification of these high-risk states in a first-degree relative is important. Antithrombin deficiency is the most thrombogenic thrombophilic state, and specialized advice for this condition should be sought from a haematologist. The precise risk will depend on the antithrombin level and whether the defect is qualitative or quantitative; antithrombin infusions might be required during delivery.

The acute management options include anticoagulation with a LMWH (e.g. enoxaparin, 1 mg/kg body weight subcutaneously twice daily), full-length support stockings on both legs and analgesia. Assessment of fetal well-being with CTG could be indicated; if labour seems imminent, a cervical assessment must be performed. Warfarin is absolutely contraindicated because it crosses the placenta and anti-coagulates the fetus, carrying a risk of fetal haemorrhage; its half-life is too long to enable safe management of delivery.

The management plan for labour is to stop anticoagulation for the minimum amount of time possible, maintain hydration (possibly with an intravenous crystalloid infusion) and keep mobility unrestricted. Regardless of the mother's current wishes for regional analgesia, this option should be kept open, especially in a primiparous woman, so that unexpected obstetric problems in labour can be managed safely and without recourse to general anaesthesia, which itself increases immo-bility and infection, and thus the risk of thrombosis. Women who have had several deliveries before without regional blockade might feel confi-dent in their ability to undergo labour without it, but even they cannot predict unexpected obstetric complications; these women also have an increased risk of postpartum haemorrhage, which is more easily managed if anticoagulation has been appropriately suspended. Most anaesthetists will not insert an epidural within 24 hours of a treatment dose of a LMWH, which could pose a problem if spontaneous onset of labour occurs shortly after administration of a dose. Women must be advised not to inject if they have any sense that labour is starting, but instead to attend the hospital for an assessment. As a result of this concern, alternative options might be considered, including changing to UH, inducing labour or performing a planned Caesarean section. Each option has distinct pros and cons, as follows:

UH – this drug was the standard treatment in pregnancy before the development of LMWHs. However, its use is cumbersome because it requires continuous intravenous infusion in high doses and regular monitoring to adjust the dose. Full anticoagulation with an activated partial thromboplastin time (APTT) twice control is often difficult to achieve. By comparison, LMWH has a standard weight-dependent dose, with twice-daily self-administration by the patient, and does not require dose monitoring. However, UH has a shorter half-life so an epidural can usually be sited within 4 hours of discontinuing the infu-sion; it is also readily reversed with protamine sulphate if obstetric haemorrhage or emergency Caesarean are required.

Induction of labour – this offers some control of when labour com-mences, so that the woman does not enter labour after injecting heparin. However, if the cervix is unfavourable and prostaglandin (PG) is required, great care must be taken to ensure that dehydration, immo-bility and pelvic vein trauma from repeated vaginal assessment are avoided while induction is taking place. Less than 50% of primiparous women are likely to deliver within 24 hours of starting a PGE_2 induc-tion. In a grandmultiparous woman, PGE_2 induction itself poses several maternal and fetal risk factors, including haemorrhage, and so it is usually avoided. It is unlikely, therefore, that PGE_2 induction would offer many benefits to this patient. However, there might be a place for serial cervical assessments and sweeps, which would enable monitoring of the progress of the cervix and provide an indication of when a simple ARM, and possibly Syntocinon, induction might be feasible. Ideally, labour will not occur within the first week, because this is the approximate time the clot takes to stabilize and the risk of extension or embolism takes to pass, and therefore it is best not to commence induction immediately in this patient.

Planned Caesarean section – as already discussed, LSCS is associated with an increased risk of thrombosis. However, if the likelihood of a vaginal delivery is estimated to be low, a planned Caesarean section is likely to be safer than an emergency Caesarean section, and so should be considered. In this patient, ideally LSCS should be performed at least 39 weeks' gestation, to ensure that the clot is as stable as possible, and LSCS should be avoided while the leg remains clinically painful and swollen. If elective LSCS is decided on, the evening dose of LMWH should be omitted; the period of "nil by mouth" should be kept to the minimum accepted by the anaesthetist and the Caesarean should be planned for as early in the morning as possible, keeping close to the 24-hour window. Immobilization should be minimized, both before and after surgery, close attention should be paid to haemostasis and prevention of infection, and the treatment dose of LMWH should be recommenced as soon as safely possible after surgery, usually 3 hours after removal of the epidural catheter (although this will be longer if there is an increased risk of haemorrhage).

After delivery, early mobilization and hydration must be encouraged. Anticoagulation usually needs to be continued for 6 months following the event. In the puerperium, the woman can switch to warfarin if she prefers. Both LMWH and warfarin are safe during lactation and both are effective at preventing further thrombosis. LMWH has the advantage of stable dosing and does not require dose monitoring. Warfarin is taken orally, but has a wide therapeutic dose range that can vary within a patient. Therefore, it is important to monitor the INR closely, to avoid accidental overdose (with the risk of haemorhage) or underdose (with the risk of recurrence). This usually entails hospital- based blood tests two to three times weekly initially and then one to two times weekly once the therapeutic window is achieved. For many women, the initial attraction of an oral medication is counterbalanced by the possibility of side effects and need for frequent hospital visits while caring for a newborn baby.

Once treatment is complete, it is essential that future care is planned. Oestrogen-containing contraception must be avoided, as should other high-risk scenarios, such as prolonged immobility, surgery and long-haul flights; smoking should be stopped and a weight-reduction programme started, if required. There should be a low threshold for thromboprophylaxis if a high-risk situation is unavoidable. The thrombophilia screen should be completed, if not already performed, and a plan for management in future pregnancies should be made. If this was a first thromboembolic event in a woman with no family history, a negative thrombophilia screen and absence of other major and unavoidable risk factors, the usual advice for a subsequent pregnancy would be to take aspirin (75 mg/day) from conception and a thromboprophylactic dose of LMWH (e.g. enoxaparin, 40 mg/day) for 6 weeks from delivery. All other women must start a thromboprophylactic dose of LMWH as soon as they know they are pregnant until the baby is 6 weeks old.

4.8 JAUNDICE

What are the most common causes of jaundice in pregnancy? How would you differentiate them?

Model Answer

Jaundice could be due to a cause co-incidental to the pregnancy or to a pregnancy-specific condition. Worldwide, the most common cause of jaundice in pregnancy is acute viral hepatitis. Other relatively common causes are acute cholecystitis, drug abuse (paracetamol and alcohol), haemolysis (e.g. sickle cell disease or malaria) and cholestatic jaundice secondary to drug use (most commonly co-amoxyclav). Pregnancy-specific causes of jaundice include obstetric cholestasis, AFLP, HELLP syndrome, pre-eclampsia, in which jaundice is rare before 20 weeks' gestation, and HG, in which jaundice can occur in the first half of pregnancy.

The cause of jaundice can usually be established by taking a thorough history, performing a careful examination, ordering appropriate investigations and then logically piecing it all together.

The gestational age should be established: if the woman is in the first half of pregnancy, it is much less likely that the jaundice is due to a pregnancy-specific cause. In the history, pruritus would point towards obstetric cholestasis or the less common autoimmune conditions of primary biliary cirrhosis or chronic active hepatitis; acute viral hepatitis and AFLP can also cause pruritus. Epigastric or right upper quadrant pain occurs in HELLP syndrome, AFLP and pre-eclampsia, in addition to biliary colic from a wide range of causes, including acute cholecystitis. Vague symptoms of malaise, flu-like illness and nausea/vomiting are nonspecific and can occur because of many causes of jaundice. Pale stools and dark urine imply cholestasis, including OC, viral hepatitis and extrahepatic biliary tract obstruction. The history might reveal previous episodes of jaundice, risk factors for liver disease, such as drug use/abuse, including alcohol and paracetamol, or a family history of liver disease (e.g. haemochromatosis, hereditary spherocytosis or Gilbert's syndrome).

On examination, the patient might be febrile, suggesting a viral hepatitis, acute cholecystitis or even AFLP. There may be hypertension and proteinuria, supporting one of the liver disorders in the spectrum of hypertensive diseases of pregnancy. Excoriation supports the symptom of pruritus; hepatomegaly, splenomegaly, ascites, lymphadenopathy and signs of chronic liver disease must be sought. However, be aware that spider naevi and palmar erythema are common in pregnancy and usually reflect the hyperoestrogenic state of pregnancy rather than chronic liver dysfunction. Intrauterine growth restriction occurs in the hypertensive disorders of pregnancy, but it is not expected with obstetric cholestasis or other acute illnesses resulting in jaundice.

Liver function tests, including serum albumin, clotting time and bile salt levels should be performed, in addition to a full blood count and film (because haemolysis can result in jaundice). In cases where haemolysis is a possibility, it is helpful to determine whether bilirubin is unconjugated (jaundice due to excess breakdown of haemoglobin, e.g. sickle cell disease, hereditary spherocytosis and HELLP syndrome or reduced ability to conjugate bilirubin e.g. Gilbert's syndrome) or conjugated (jaundice due to intrahepatic or extrahepatic causes). Renal function incorporating urate and blood glucose must also be measured. These results alone will not usually confirm a diagnosis, but can point to an intrahepatic or extrahepatic clinical picture, depending on the relative elevation of the transaminases, alkaline phosphatase and gamma glutamyl transferase levels. A prolonged prothrombin time and hypoglycaemia might suggest acute failure of hepatic synthesis; hypoalbuminaemia suggests chronic synthetic dysfunction, but also occurs with heavy proteinuria (e.g. pre-eclampsia). Remember that alkaline phosphatase increases threefold by the third trimester of normal pregnancy because of placental production of a heat-stable isoenzyme. It might be helpful to ask the laboratory to heat treat the sample to 60°C for 10 minutes and then rerun the assay: the difference between the first and the second measurements represents the level of liver isoenzyme. Relatively minor elevations in transaminases can occur in end-stage liver disease, where there is massive hepatocellular damage and few surviving hepatocytes. Elevated bile salt levels are a sensitive marker for cholestasis but are not pathognomonic of one particular liver disease, nor are they an essential diagnostic criterion for any condition.

A viral hepatitis screen for hepatitis A, B and C, and in relevant areas of the world hepatitis E, in addition to Epstein-Barr virus and cytomegalovirus, should be requested because this will provide information regarding an infective process; human immunodeficiency virus (HIV) screening should be considered. A liver autoantibody screen, incorporating antimitochondrial, anti-smooth muscle and antinuclear cytoplasmic antibodies, should be considered if primary biliary cirrhosis, autoimmune chronic active hepatitis or sclerosing cholangitis form part of the differential diagnosis. Liver ultrasound can be helpful, especially if extrahepatic obstruction is suspected (e.g. cholelithiasis) or to diagnose features compatible with chronic liver disease, such as hepatomegaly, splenomegaly, focal lesions, general parenchymal disease, portal and hepatic vein patency or the presence of varices, detection of ascites and lymphadenopathy. The presence of liver steatosis is insufficiently specific or sensitive to clarify the diagnosis. Liver biopsy might be considered, especially if coagulation is normal, the diagnosis, and therefore management, is in doubt: this is particularly true if the woman is preterm and delivery of the fetus is being considered, because not all conditions will improve postnatally.

A multidisciplinary approach is likely to be needed, either to help determination of the cause of jaundice or to help ongoing management.

4.9 CHICKEN POX

You are phoned by a GP. He has just seen a woman who is 12 weeks' pregnant, and whose son has chickenpox. What advice should the pregnant woman be given, and why? What are the risks of chickenpox in pregnancy?

Model Answer

At least 90% of adults born in the UK will be immune to chickenpox. Among those who are unaware of previous exposure, approaching 90% will also be immune. If, however, she has only recently arrived in the UK from tropical or subtropical regions, she is much less likely to be immune (around 50%). The easiest way to establish immunity is to ask whether she recollects having chickenpox. If she was brought up in America or Japan, she might have had immunization against chickenpox as part of the national immunization programme: she should be asked about this too.

If she has not had chickenpox previously nor been vaccinated against it, her GP should review her records for evidence of previous testing, because some hospitals screen pregnant women who are unaware of exposure for chickenpox immunity. Assuming there is no record of immunity, there are two options. First, if she has had blood taken recently, for example for her booking blood tests, the laboratory might have a stored sample that could be tested. If stored serum is not available, 10 ml of clotted blood should be sent urgently to the laboratory, marked "urgent, pregnant, close contact with chickenpox – please measure VZV IgG". Most laboratories should be able to provide a result within 24–48 hours if they are aware of the urgency of the sample. Assuming that an enzyme-linked immunoassay or indirect immunofluorescence test is used, there is a high degree of sensitivity.

In the interim, she should avoid close contact with pregnant women who have not had chickenpox and neonates. She should also report immediately if she develops clinical symptoms of chickenpox, so that aciclovir can be considered (see below). In addition, her son should see his GP to confirm that his rash is typical of varicella.

If she is not immune to chickenpox, she should have varicella zoster immunoglobulin (VZIG) as soon as possible, up to 10 days after the *first* contact with chickenpox, and only if this is before the rash appears; VZIG is of no benefit once chickenpox has developed. She should be asked whether she has had any other recent contact with chickenpox: for example, does she know where her son contracted chickenpox, and was she significantly exposed at the same time? This reduces the risk of chickenpox from a household contact by about 40%. However, only 27% of women remain uninfected: 25% have a subclinical infection, 32% have mild disease, and the remainder have severe disease. There is also some evidence that VZIG reduces the occurrence and severity of fetal infection, fetal varicella syndrome and varicella of the newborn. Other groups of patients who are at increased risk from chickenpox include those who are immunocompromised (including those taking immunosuppressive agents, such as steroids and symptomatic HIV-positive individuals). Her medical history should be reviewed to ensure she is not at higher risk than usual for pregnancy.

The risks of chickenpox relate to fetal, neonatal and maternal issues. If chickenpox occurs before 13 weeks' gestation, the risk of fetal varicella syndrome is 0.4%, and if chickenpox occurs between 13 weeks' and 20 weeks' gestation the risk is 2% [9]; occasional cases have been reported after 20 weeks' gestation [10], but none beyond 28 weeks' gestation. The fetal problems are because of herpes zoster reactivation *in utero* rather than fetal chickenpox per se, and occur mostly at less than 20 weeks' gestation because the fetus lacks the cell-mediated immunity required to control reactivation until this gestation. The wide range of anomalies is due to tissue and neuronal damage by secondary reactivation of the virus in latently infected dorsal root ganglia, and may be external or internal. Typical features include skin scarring in a dermatomal distribution, limb hypoplasia, neurological abnormalities (including bowel and bladder dysfunction, microcephaly, mental retardation and cortical atrophy) and eye defects (microphthalmia, cataracts and chorioretinitis) and reflect the damage to the fetal nervous system. Ultrasound assessment of the fetus might detect polyhydramnios, hyperechogenic bowel, hyperechogenic foci in the liver or hydrops fetalis, but these will not be apparent for several weeks after maternal viraemia. Serial scans should be organized. There is little place for invasive procedures: although amniocentesis in the first half of pregnancy will detect varicella zoster virus (VZV) DNA in about 8% cases, less than 50% of these fetuses will be affected. The incidence of fetal viraemia increases with the length of gestation, but does not reflect the risk to the fetus, because of the increasing maturity of its immune system.

Varicella of the newborn (previously referred to as "congenital varicella") is due to vertical transmission. It is particularly severe if the mother has chickenpox 7 days before or 2 days after delivery, because protective maternal antibodies, which could cross the placenta, have not formed but fetal viraemia is possible. Neonatal mortality may be as high as 30%. Neonatal infection occurs in about 60% of babies whose mothers are infected in the 28 days before delivery, but is more likely to be subclinical if maternal infection occurs further from delivery (because of the ameliorating effect of maternal antibodies). Herpes zoster could occur in the first few months of life in babies whose mothers have chickenpox during pregnancy, but this is usually benign.

Chickenpox in adults can be more severe than in children, and there is some evidence that chickenpox in pregnancy increases the risk of complications further, especially in the later stages of pregnancy. Pneumonitis occurs in about 8% of pregnant women: she should be warned to report early if the symptoms of pneumonitis, including cough, tachypnoea, dyspnoea, haemoptysis and chest pain, occur, especially if she is at increased risk because of smoking or chronic lung disease. Other complications of chickenpox include secondary skin sepsis, hepatitis, haemorrhagic rash and encephalitis; mortality is estimated at 1–2%.

Aciclovir is thought to reduce the severity and duration of chickenpox in the pregnant woman, but only if it is given within 24 hours of the onset of the rash: she must be told to make immediate contact if chickenpox occurs and provided with details of who to contact at weekends and where to attend. Aciclovir is now believed to be safe in pregnancy. The aciclovir registry for reporting use of this drug in pregnancy closed in 1998, after almost 1300 cases were reported, with no evidence of adverse fetal effects. It is recommended that oral aciclovir (800 mg five times daily) is taken for 7 days by women who present within 24 hours of the onset of the rash and are beyond 20 weeks' gestation. In women who are less than 20 weeks' gestation, as this woman is, aciclovir should be offered rather than recommended, because of theoretical concerns relating to teratogenesis.

Intravenous aciclovir (10 mg/kg body weight three times daily) should be used if varicella pneumonitis develops or there is evidence of disease progression, such as continued cropping of the rash beyond day 6, reappearance of fever after day 6, thrombocytopenia, hepatitis or skin sepsis. If she does develop chickenpox, she should be assessed every 24–48 hours to ensure that any early signs of complications are detected.

REFERENCES

1. Millar LK et al. Low birth weight and pre-eclampsia in pregnancies complicated by hyperthyroidism. *Obstet Gynecol* 1994; **84:** 946–9.
2. Momotani N et al. Effects of Propylthiouracil and methimazole on fetal thyroid status in mothers with Graves' hyperthyroidism. *J Clin Endocrin Metab* 1997; **82:** 3633–6.
3. Wing DA et al. A comparison of Propylthiouracil versus methimazole in the treatment of hyperthyroidism in pregnancy. *Am J Obstet Gynecol* 1994; **170:** 90–5.
4. Momotani N et al. Maternal hyperthyroidism and congenital malformation in the offspring. *Clin Endocrin* 1984; **20:** 695–700.
5. Hershman JM. Role of human chorionic gonadotropin as a thyroid stimulator. *J Clin Endo Metab* 1992; **74:** 258–9.
6. Chowdhury TA et al. A toxic testicle. *Lancet* 2000; **355:** 2046.
7. Rodien P et al. Familial gestational hyperthyroidism caused by a mutant thyrotropin receptor hypersensitive to human chorionic gonadotropin. *New Engl J Med* 1998; **339:** 1823–6.
8. Confidential Enquiry into Maternal And Child Health (CEMACH). Type 1 and type 2 diabetes in pregnancy, 2005.
9. Enders G, Miller E, Cradock-Watson J et al. Consequences of varicella and herpes zoster in pregnancy: a prospective study of 1739 pregnancies. *Lancet* 1994; **343:** 1548–51.
10. Drugs and Therapeutics Bulletin, 'Chickenpox, pregnancy and the newborn' September 2005.

Chapter 5
Case Studies

5.1 SICKLE CELL DISEASE

Ms A was a 28 year old woman in her second pregnancy (she had one previous termination of pregnancy) who booked-in at 19 weeks' gestation. She was known to have sickle cell disease (specifically sickle cell anaemia [HbSS]), and her last crisis had occurred 3 years before this pregnancy.

Her booking bloods were unremarkable. Her blood pressure and haemoglobin (Hb) concentration were recorded as 90/60 mmHg and 8.1 g/dl, respectively, with an mean cell volume (MCV) of 87 fL. At this visit, she was commenced on penicillin (250 mg/day), folate (5 mg/day) and 4-weekly growth scans were organized.

Her first admission to hospital was a month later (at 23 weeks' gestation), when she was admitted for 6 days with a crisis (pain in her back), which was possibly precipitated by a urinary tract infection. She was initially treated with intravenous cefuroxime and thereafter with oral clarithromycin. She received a 3-unit blood transfusion, which co-incided with a symptomatic improvement.

Her second admission (for 12 days) occurred 2 weeks later (at 25 weeks' gestation); again, she was treated for a crisis. She required another 3-unit blood transfusion because her Hb concentration had fallen to 6.8 g/dl. She required an opiate patient-controlled analgesia (PCA) and was treated with intravenous fluids, cefuroxime, metronidazole and flucloxacillin.

During her third admission (at 30 weeks' gestation for 7 days), when she had chest pain and blood-stained sputum, she was treated with intravenous antibiotics and a therapeutic dose (1 mg/kg body weight/twice daily) of enoxaparin (until a ventilation/perfusion [V/Q] lung scan was negative). Her blood cultures and sputum were negative and a further 2-unit transfusion was required.

Her fourth admission occurred within days of discharge from the hospital. Her symptoms included worsening chest pain and shortness of breath. On examination, there were crepitations and dullness in the base of the right lung. She was treated with further intravenous antibiotics for presumptive community-acquired pneumonia, but she also had another inconclusive V/Q lung scan and was thus recommenced on a therapeutic dose of enoxaparin. She was discharged at 33 weeks' gestation with oral antibiotics (clarithromycin, flucloxacillin, cephadroxil and nystatin) and enoxaparin.

In total, she had seven ultrasound scans, which showed a small baby (growth on the third centile), with normal liquor volume and umbilical Doppler scan.

At 38 weeks' gestation, she underwent induction of labour and received two doses of vaginal prostaglandin. However, fetal distress necessitated a Caesarean section under general anaesthetic. She delivered a 2.72 kg baby, with a pH of 7.22 and Apgar score of 5 and 9 at 1 minute and 5 minutes, respectively.

Discussion

Sickle cell disease results when there is a variant of the beta-globin chain (a one amino-acid substitution of valine with glutamine). In times of crises, which can be precipitated by a number of factors (e.g. hypoxia, infection, cold, acidosis and dehydration), the red cell takes on a characteristic, distorted shape. Because of this rigidity, it tends to block small vessels, producing vaso-occlusive symptoms (pain) and even infarction.

This patient last had a crisis 3 years before this pregnancy, but during this pregnancy she developed three crises. This reflects the increased complication rate and increased tendency to crises in women with sickle cell disease who fall pregnant. They suffer from chronic anaemia (Ms A's booking Hb concentration was 8.1 g/dl), because of chronic haemolysis, which is often asymptomatic. This is because of the low affinity of sickle Hb (HbS) for oxygen, which facilitates oxygen delivery to the tissues.

The possible effects of sickle cell disease on the pregnancy were also reflected by the small, growth-restricted baby who could not tolerate the stress of labour. This necessitated a Caesarean section. Unexplained stillbirth is not uncommon in these patients because of both impaired oxygen supply and sickling infarcts in the placental circulation. Therefore, it is the unit policy to offer induction to all women with sickle cell disease at 38 weeks' gestation.

This pregnancy was complicated by frequent admissions with crises and chest infections. It is often difficult to distinguish between pneumonia, sickle chest syndrome and pulmonary embolism because these conditions share similar signs and symptoms (tachypnoea, pleuritic chest pain and leucocytosis) [1]. Early recourse to antibiotics and rehydration is important to prevent further morbidity and mortality because most deaths are due to massive sickling following an infection, which leads to a pulmonary embolism [2].

Ms A received three blood transfusions during this pregnancy. Letsky [2] reported that the only consistently successful way to reduce the incidence of complications from sickling is regular blood transfusion at approximately 6-weekly intervals. This aims to dilute the existing HbS, and by raising the Hb concentration, thus reduce the stimulus to the bone marrow to produce more defective cells. This policy does, however, expose the patient to the risks of multiple transfusions (i.e. alloimmunization and infection) and it does not have universal acceptance.

At present, there is no effective long-term method of reducing the lability of red cells in vivo. There is no evidence to support the use of alkalis, hyperbaric oxygen, vasodilators, plasma expanders or anticoagulation once the crisis is established. The best approach is meticulous care and supportive therapy with adequate fluids, analgesia and treatment of possible infection. Prophylactic antibiotics (e.g. penicillin) are used because patients with sickle cell disease often have a nonfunctioning spleen and penicillin affords protection against pneumococcal septicaemia.

5.2 HYPONATRAEMIA

Ms B was a 29 year old primigravid who booked-in at 16 weeks' gestation. Her booking bloods were unremarkable. Her blood pressure and Hb concentration were recorded as 100/60 mmHg and 11.2 g/dl, respectively.

She had seven uneventful antenatal visits throughout which she had a normal blood pressure and no abnormalities were found in her urine.

She self-presented at term in spontaneous labour, and in the ensuing 48 hours, despite a prolonged latent phase, she delivered a 3.54 kg infant with Apgar scores of 8 and 9 at 1 and 5 mins respectively. This was facilitated by an instrumental delivery in theatre. She required an epidural and Syntocinon for the last 12 hours of her labour. The Syntocinon was infused (as per protocol) at an increasing rate of 1 mu/min and titrated to her contractions.

It was noted that she had only passed 70 ml of urine 5 hours after the insertion of the epidural and urinary catheter, despite receiving 1500 ml of intravenous and oral fluids. The catheter was flushed and a 500 ml fluid challenge was given. Her vital signs were stable. After 2 hours (at 7.30 a.m.), a baseline renal function test was performed (Table 5.1).

TABLE 5.1. Serial urea and electrolytes

Time	7.30 a.m.	12.30 p.m.	8.10 p.m.	5.30 a.m.
Sodium, mmol/l	124	121	131	140
Creatinine, μmol/l	96	131	110	81
Urea, mmol/l	4.7	5.4	5.7	4.6
Serum osmolality		262		
Bicarbonate, mmol/l	19	17	19	22

Because of continuing oliguria, a further fluid challenge was administered at 10.30 a.m. Her serum osmolality was 262 mOsm/kg (normal range, 275–285 mOsm/kg) and her urine osmolality was 338 mOsm/kg.

Further blood testing performed before ventouse delivery (at 12.30 p.m.) showed worsening renal function and hyponatraemia (Table 5.1).

With a presumptive diagnosis of "water intoxication" secondary to Syntocinon administration, Ms B received treatment postoperatively with fluid restriction (500 ml/12 hours). In the following 8 hours, a massive diuresis occurred (6.5 l). By 17 hours postdelivery, her renal function had significantly improved (Table 1) and she was discharged home a day later.

Discussion

Hyponatraemia is the commonest electrolyte disturbance seen in a general hospital population, occurring in 1% of all patients. It is defined as a decrease in serum sodium concentration below the normal range (136–145 mmol/l), usually indicative of hypo-osmolality of body fluid due to an excess of water relative to solute.

It has two principle causes, as follows:

1. Sodium depletion in excess of water or replacement of sodium losses with water alone, for example in gastrointestinal and third-space losses, sweating and dialysis/renal failure.
2. Dilutional hyponatraemia occurs if the water intake is in excess of its output and usually implies impaired excretion. This occurs in cases ranging from inappropriate secretion of antidiuretic hormone (ADH) to those resulting from neuroendocrine, adrenal or pituitary insufficiency.

The causes of the syndrome of inappropriate secretion of ADH (SIADH) can broadly be divided into those secondary to malignancy (tumours of the lung, pancreas or duodenum), central nervous system disorders (meningitis, head injury or haemorrhage), chest disease (tuberculosis or pneumonia) or metabolic disease (porphyria).

Well-known complications of oxytocin include overstimulation of the myometrium, resulting in tetanic contractions, fetal hypoxia or occasionally uterine rupture. A lesser-known side effect is that it has an ADH-like effect, leading to suppression of diuresis and features including concentrated urine, hyponatraemia and low plasma osmolality with no apparent dehydration or oedema. "Water intoxication", as it was called, was first reported in 1962 by Liggins [3]. This complication occurred in women receiving large doses of oxytocin, most commonly in those having midtrimester termination of pregnancy or the induction of premature labour associated with fetal death in utero. It usually involved large amounts of oxytocin in electrolyte-free solutions administered over an extended time period, which resulted in severe electrolyte derangements, convulsions, coma and even death [4].

The pathogenesis involves progressive hyponatraemia and fluid shifts from the extravascular to the intravascular compartment, with resultant cerebral oedema. Transplacental passage can occur with similar derangements in neonatal biochemistry [5]. Convulsions are unlikely unless the fluid input exceeds output by >3 l in 24 hours, and are, therefore, uncommon following oxytocin-induced labour at term.

This patient, however, was given low doses of Syntocinon (1 mu/min and then 2 mu/min) over a moderate time period (7 hours). Even allowing for the small incremental dosage increases that occurred with the step-up Syntocinon regimen, a low total dose of oxytocin was infused. In retrospect, the two fluid challenges she received probably exacerbated hyponatraemia.

Current labour ward protocols limit the use of oxytocin in terms of concentration, duration of administration and type of additional fluids. Stratton et al. [6] showed that patients who received co-infusions of dextrose solution had significantly lower sodium levels compared with patients who received electrolyte infusions (normal saline). Most units use Hartmann's solution or normal saline for oxytocin administration.

Correct use of the partogram limits the duration of the active phase of labour; thus, rarely do patients "labour" for >24 hours in hospital, minimizing oxytocin infusion times and risks.

A literature review using Medline revealed a predominance of cases in the early 1970s and 1980s, with a paucity of new reports, suggesting that water intoxication secondary to oxytocin administration rarely occurs nowadays. However, clinicians should remain vigilant to the possibility.

The primary treatment is recognition of the underlying cause (stopping oxytocin) and thereafter restricting intake to 1000–1500 ml/ 24 hours.

This might seem an illogical step because of oliguria, but if the diagnosis is correct, it will result in rapid improvement. Similar to pre-eclampsia, the use of repeated blind fluid challenges should be avoided in the labouring or postpartum patient unless volume depletion or blood loss is suspected.

5.3 ISCHAEMIC HEART DISEASE

Ms C was a 32 year old caucasian woman. She was para 0 + 1, having had a fetal loss at 23 weeks' gestation 1 year previously. She attended the obstetric medicine clinic at 7 weeks' gestation, having been referred by her general practitioner (GP).

In her past medical history, she had had a myocardial infarction with coronary artery stenting aged 27, with ongoing angina, hypercholesterolaemia, hypertension, asthma, oesophageal reflux and chronic back pain.

She had conceived while taking aspirin, isosorbide mononitrate, glyceryl trinitrate (GTN) spray, ramipril, simvastatin, montelukast, omeprazole, codeine phosphate, diazepam, and beclomethasone and salbutamol inhalers.

She was a current smoker of 40 cigarettes/day and was homeless and living in a hostel. During investigation of the previous intrauterine death, raised anticardiolipin antibodies were detected on two occasions >8 weeks apart. She had an initial booking ultrasound that showed a twin pregnancy.

There was a long discussion regarding her medication, and after appropriate counselling, she was advised to stop simvastatin, ramipril and omeprazole and to reduce codeine phosphate and diazepam as much as possible. She was also referred to a smoking cessation clinic. Her angiotensin-converting enzyme (ACE) inhibitor was changed to methyldopa and omeprazole was changed to ranitidine. She was commenced on enoxaparin (40 mg once daily) and folic acid (5 mg/day), which was to be continued throughout the pregnancy. She was understandably very anxious regarding the pregnancy.

She returned for her booking appointment at 10 weeks' gestation. A repeat scan showed no fetal heart in one twin. Booking bloods were taken, plus urea, electrolytes and urate measurements, which were normal. Repeat anticardiolipin antibodies remained elevated.

A management plan was made for the pregnancy. She was to be seen in the obstetric medicine clinic once per fortnight for blood pressure measurement and urinalysis, and monitoring of her angina symptoms, which she was at times reluctant to admit to. She was offered serum screening at 16 weeks' gestation.

At her request she was commenced on high-dose vitamin C (1 g/day) and vitamin E (400 iu/day) [7]. A fetal anomaly scan was organized at 18 weeks' gestation, with maternal uterine artery Doppler estimation. Growth scans were planned from 24 weeks' gestation and delivery was planned by elective Caesarean section at 38–39 weeks' gestation.

The pregnancy progressed uneventfully until 20 weeks' gestation. The fetal anomaly scan showed no anomalies in the fetus but there was bilateral notching on the uterine artery Doppler scan. She managed to cut down smoking to two to three cigarettes/day and the social work department was involved regarding her housing situation. She became increasingly stressed and complained of increasing angina. Her isosorbide mononitrate was increased. Her anxiety grew further around the time of her previous loss.

Growth scans estimated that the baby was growing between the 5th and the 50th centiles.

The woman complained of further episodes of angina, even on minimal exertion and despite using her GTN spray. Her isosorbide mononitrate was further increased. An echocardiogram was performed at 36 weeks' gestation. This showed a normal ejection fraction, with good systolic function. An electrocardiogram (ECG) was normal. She was reviewed by the obstetric anaesthetic team.

The planned elective Caesarean section was carried out at >38 weeks' gestation.

Her low-molecular-weight heparin (LMWH) was stopped on the day before the planned surgery. A combined spinal epidural was used for analgesia and the Caesarean section was uncomplicated, with 400 ml blood loss. She delivered a live male infant, with a birth weight of 2.95 kg.

Ms C recovered well from the Caesarean section and wished to breastfeed. Unfortunately, varying advice was given over the safety of her medication in breastfeeding. Breastfeeding did not establish easily and she bottle fed her son from 6 days of age. She continued on enoxaparin (40 mg once daily) for 6 weeks postpartum. Her ACE inhibitor and statin were restarted. At 6 weeks postpartum, both mother and baby were well. She was considering a Mirena intrauterine system (IUS) for future contraception, although she was not currently with her partner. She was counselled regarding the risks of a further pregnancy.

Discussion

This was a high-risk pregnancy in a woman with extensive medical and social problems. She had significant risk factors and ischaemic heart disease, with ongoing symptoms, despite her young age. It was felt that her previous myocardial infarction was due to ischaemic heart disease in the presence of underlying risk factors of hypercholesterolaemia, hypertension and smoking rather than because of arterial thrombosis from her antiphospholipid antibody syndrome (APS). APS (late fetal loss in the presence of raised anticardiolipin antibodies) also posed risks to the pregnancy, which could be reduced by LMWH and low-dose aspirin. She conceived while receiving a large number of drugs, for which there are minimal data on use in pregnancy and breastfeeding.

There is very little literature on women with ischaemic heart disease in pregnancy because until recently this was rare in women of childbearing age [8,9].

The continued use of ACE inhibitors in pregnancy has been associated with foetotoxicity (fetal renal failure and renal dysgenesis, hypotension, oligohydramnios, pulmonary hypoplasia and hypocalvaria). The risks are greatest during the second and third trimester [10]. Women should change to an alternative antihypertensive pre pregnancy. ACE inhibitors are safe to use while breastfeeding, but as this case illustrates, this is not widely appreciated.

A recent multicentre study showed no increase in anomalies in the fetus exposed to omeprazole in the first trimester [11]. Montelukast has little safety data in human pregnancy; however, animal studies have been reassuring (it has been categorized as US Food and Drug Administration [FDA] pregnancy category B). In cases of severe asthma requiring the use of montelukast during pregnancy, many clinicians continue this drug because the risks to the fetus of poorly controlled asthma in the mother outweigh any potential risks of the drug.

APS has been extensively studied in pregnancy and there is good evidence for the benefit of the use of both low-dose aspirin and LMWH in these women, both to prevent early miscarriage and to prevent thrombosis [12]. There is less evidence that it reduces the risk of intrauterine growth restriction (IUGR) or late still birth.

5.4 CARDIAC TRANSPLANT

Mrs D was a 33 year old para 0 + 1 who attended for prepregnancy counselling with her husband and mother. She had received a cardiac transplant 10 years previously at the age of 24 following multiple myocardial infarcts caused by thromboemboli. Postmyocardial infarction, her left ventricular ejection fraction was 13% on an echocardiogram. She was, therefore, placed on the cardiac transplant waiting list and received a transplant 5 months after her initial myocardial infarction. She had three episodes of rejection in the early period following her transplant, but these were all mild. She had not had any other episodes of rejection.

She had been followed-up regularly at the transplant centre and remained very well.

Her most recent coronary angiogram, performed a year earlier, was normal with no evidence of allograft coronary artery disease. She had also had an echocardiogram showing mild left-ventricular hypertrophy, but with good function. The right ventricle was normal. She had a thickened aortic valve with mild aortic regurgitation and a mildly thickened mitral valve with mild mitral regurgitation. An ECG showed right bundle branch block.

Her current medication was as follows:

Ciclosporin A, 125 mg twice daily.
Azathioprine, 75 mg once daily.
Prednisolone, 5 mg once daily.

Atorvastatin, 10 mg at night had been stopped in preparation for pregnancy.

A thrombophilia screen was negative and prepregnancy serum creatinine was 116 μmol/l.

A review of the literature was performed in order to advise her and she was given a follow-up appointment for further discussion.

At her follow-up appointment, Mrs D reported a positive pregnancy test. Her booking blood pressure was 140/84 mmHg at 8 weeks' gestation. Urinalysis showed 4+ blood, 1+ protein (she reported some PV bleeding.) Baseline electrolytes, urate level and ciclosporin A levels were performed. A 24-hour urine collection for creatinine clearance and total protein estimation and an MSU were also performed. Mrs D was commenced on aspirin (75 mg/day) and folate (5 mg/day) to be continued throughout the pregnancy. She had a normal nuchal translucency and first trimester scan. Maternal uterine artery Doppler studies were arranged for 24 weeks' gestation and showed a prediastolic "notch" and persistent high-resistance waveform predictive of subsequent pre-eclampsia, IUGR or placental abruption.

Mrs D had an uneventful antenatal course but delivered by emergency Caesarean section at 36 weeks' gestation in another unit following an abruption. Mother and baby are well.

Discussion

The literature describes 57 pregnancies in 41 women postcardiac transplantation. The overall reported incidence of miscarriage is 14%, with a preterm delivery rate at <37 weeks' gestation of 30% and an incidence of pre-eclampsia of 17.5% [13,14,15].

The main clinical issues for Mrs D were as follows:

Medication – there is evidence that ciclosporin A causes IUGR in women who become pregnant while taking this drug. Therefore, the lowest dose possible should be the aim. However, the maternal risks of voluntarily ceasing the medication are very high and in the literature three reported maternal deaths followed voluntary cessation of immunosuppressants.

Renal impairment – baseline bloods were normal, with the exception of serum creatinine, which was raised (105 μmol/l), although this represented an appropriate pregnancy-related fall compared with the preconception level (116 μmol/l). Raised serum creatinine might have been due, in part, to her excess muscle mass (she was an avid weight-training enthusiast), in which case it should fall following cessation of excessive exercise as she was advised, or it could have been due to a degree of nephrotoxicity from ciclosporin A. If it was due to nephrotoxicity, the development of pre-eclampsia was more likely. This was the rationale behind starting aspirin therapy.

Measurement of resting pulse rate was important because transplanted hearts are denervated and thus there is always a resting tachycardia. It is important to document the patient's normal heart rate. She should also have an ECG because there might be minor abnormalities, which are normal for her, and it is important to record this.

In the largest series of heart-transplant recipients with subsequent pregnancy, maternal survival was 71% at 7.5 years [15]. In all other case series, the mothers were described as healthy in the immediate postpartum period. Reduced maternal survival while the child is still young was also discussed with the couple.

This largest series reported 47 pregnancies in 35 women: 6 pregnancies ended in miscarriage and 6 ended in therapeutic abortion. The incidence of preterm delivery at <37 weeks' gestation was 43% and the mean birth weight was 2543 g ± 696 g. There were no structural abnormalities reported in the infants. The incidence of pre-eclampsia was 20% and allograft vasculopathy was 24%, which is not higher than would be expected in any 1 year in a heart-transplant patient who was not pregnant.

Nine women in this series died and, importantly, three of these women had ceased taking their immunosuppressant therapy because of concerns regarding the fetus.

5.5 POSTPARTUM ECLAMPSIA

Ms E was a 22 year old primigravid woman. She attended for routine booking at 12 weeks' gestation, at which time all investigations were normal. She was fit and well, with no significant past medical or family history. Her booking blood pressure was 96/50 mmHg, and urinalysis was negative. She received routine antenatal care and remained well throughout her pregnancy; she was normotensive with no proteinuria throughout.

At 41+3 weeks' gestation she was admitted in spontaneous labour. On admission, her blood pressure was recorded as 150/87 mmHg.

Labour progressed well, but at full dilation, following active pushing for 1 hour, the head was in a deflexed occipito-posterior position with the vertex above the ischial spines, and a decision for emergency Caesarean section was made. This was carried out uneventfully and a live male infant weighing 3.3 kg was delivered in good condition. Blood loss at the time of operation was estimated at 700 ml, with subsequent blood loss of approximately 500 ml.

On day 1 post Caesarean section, she developed abdominal distension. Her blood pressure was recorded as 121/54 mmHg. An abdominal X-ray was performed and this showed dilated loops of bowel consistent with a paralytic ileus. She was thus transferred to the high-dependency unit, where a nasogastric tube was inserted and intravenous fluids were commenced. Routine bloods were taken (Table 5.2). She was found to be anaemic, with a Hb concentration of 8.4 g/dl and was transfused with two units of red blood cells. The following day, her abdominal distension was less. Her bowels opened following an enema and there were some bowel sounds present.

On day 3 postnatally, she complained of a severe headache at midnight; her blood pressure was recorded as 185/87 mmHg and she was given 50 mg of pethidine intramuscularly because simple analgesia was inadequate. After 1 hour (on day 4 at 1 a.m.), the on-call registrar was called to see her urgently because she was having a tonic–clonic convulsion. She was given facial oxygen and a magnesium sulphate ($MgSO_4$) bolus, followed by an infusion. The convulsion terminated after 10 minutes. In retrospect, on her chart her blood pressure had been recorded as 178/81–185/90 mmHg since 5 p.m. that day. Urinalysis showed 2+ proteinuria. Electrolytes, urate, a full blood count, coagulation screen and liver function tests were checked (Table 5.2).

Her blood pressure remained stable at about 126/78 mmHg. Further bloods tests were repeated. A computed tomography (CT) brain scan was performed the following day and reported as normal. By day 5, she was feeling better and her ileus was improving. $MgSO_4$ infusion was stopped after 24 hours.

At 6 a.m. on day 6 post Caesarean section, the registrar was called urgently to see her because she was having a further tonic–clonic convulsion. She had not complained of any prodromal symptoms.

TABLE 5.2. Flow chart of Ms E's blood test results

Result		convulsion ↓	convulsion ↓				
Post-C/S	Day 2	Day 4	Day 6	Day 7	Day 8	Day 10	Day 12
Na, mmol/l	141	144	141	143	140	142	135
K, mmol/l	4.0	3.6	3.5	3.7	3.3	4.7	4.3
Urea mmol/l	2.9	4.6	7.4	10.6	12.4	9.9	5.7
Creatinine, μmol/l	60	87	176	225	264	202	117
Urate, mmol/l	0.40	0.69		0.71	0.58	0.42	
Albumin, g/l	18	19	20	22	21	25	
ALT, iu/l	7	11	8	8	7	19	
Alkaline phosphatase, iu/l	188	179	149	159	142	143	

ALT - alanine transaminase; C/S - Caesarean section; K - potassium; Na - sodium.

This convulsion terminated after 3 minutes. In retrospect, her blood pressure had been recorded as 146/99 mmHg at 3 a.m. Repeat blood tests were performed. She was commenced on atenolol, 50 mg once daily. Her blood pressure was subsequently well controlled and she had no further convulsions. However her renal function continued to deteriorate (Table 5.2).

Her abdominal distension gradually reduced and she began eating and drinking normally again. There were issues regarding bonding with the baby: Ms E showed no interest in her son and wanted her family to look after him at home. She was encouraged to have him beside her as much as possible. She had regular reviews by obstetric medicine and renal physicians. Her urine output remained excellent despite deteriorating renal function. A renal scan was performed on day 11. This was reported as showing normal kidneys of equal size, slight pelvicaliceal system dilatation, probably because of incomplete bladder emptying, and a postmicturition residual volume of 450 ml. This scan result was discussed with the urologists and she was allowed home with an in-dwelling catheter and plans for out-patient review.

Her renal function improved (Table 5.2). She was well enough to be discharged home on day 13, with the following discharge medication: ferrous sulphate ($FeSO_4$) 200 mg twice per day and atenolol (50 mg once per day).

When reviewed in the obstetric medicine clinic at 5 weeks postpartum, she was well and normotensive (110/70 mmHg), and urinalysis was clear. Her serum creatinine was 87 μmol/l. Atenolol was discontinued and GP follow-up was arranged. Urodynamic follow-up was organized by the urology department.

Discussion

With improvements in antenatal care and both improved recognition and earlier diagnosis of pre-eclampsia, in addition to earlier delivery for those with severe pre-eclampsia, there seems to have been a shift in the timing of eclampsia towards the postpartum period, perhaps increasingly >48 hours post-delivery. Of eclamptic convulsions, 44% occur postpartum.

More than one-third of women experience their first convulsion before the development of hypertension and proteinuria. In the vast majority of patients, at least one prodromal symptom is experienced. In a recent study, 87% had headache, 44% had visual symptoms, 22% had nausea or vomiting and 9% had epigastric pain [16].

Fortuitously, this woman remained an in-patient because she developed a paralytic ileus; she would otherwise have been discharged and had the convulsion at home.

Her blood pressure was elevated both in the immediate postpartum period and between her convulsions, but it remained untreated; this was probably owing, in part, to the focus on her paralytic ileus and, in part, because of being falsely reassured by the normal blood profile on day 2 [17].

Her headache, severe enough to require opiate analgesia, should have prompted further examination and investigation because it heralded her first convulsion.

Her blood pressure was markedly elevated before her second convulsion, although there were no prodromal symptoms.

MgSO$_4$ had been discontinued after 24 hours (as per protocol), and it is difficult to predict which patients will develop recurrent convulsions and require additional therapy [18].

Beware of the routine use of nonsteroidal anti-inflammatory drugs (NSAIDs) following Caesarean section. This patient received two doses of voltarol despite deteriorating renal function.

5.6 HYPEREMESIS GRAVIDARUM

Ms F was a 35 year old woman in her third pregnancy. In her first pregnancy, she had been admitted on four occasions with severe hyperemesis and needed prolonged periods of hospitalization, in addition to regular antiemetics until 33 weeks' gestation. She terminated her second pregnancy because she could not face such severe hyperemesis again.

She was previously fit and well, but in the index pregnancy, she experienced nausea and vomiting from her first missed period and presented to the hospital at 8 weeks' gestation. On examination, she was tachycardiac and had postural hypotension and ketonuria. Ms F was admitted and treated with intravenous fluids and metoclopramide, 10 mg intramuscularly three times daily. A viable intrauterine pregnancy was confirmed on ultrasound scan; she improved on the above therapy and was discharged 2 days later. In the subsequent 2 weeks, she had three further admissions with hyperemesis gravidarum (HG). On the third occasion, she was severely dehydrated, had lost 7 kg in weight and was ketotic. She was admitted, rehydrated and given regular cyclizine, 50 mg intravenously three times daily. Over the following week, she improved and was sent home with oral antiemetics, folic acid (5 mg) and thiamine hydrochloride (25 mg three times daily).

Her next admission was at 12 weeks' gestation despite regular use of oral cyclizine. She had lost a further 3 kg in weight and, again, had 4+ ketones in her urine. Investigations revealed a raised free thyroxine (fT$_4$) level, undetectable thyroid-stimulating hormone (TSH), abnormal liver function with an alanine aminotransferase (ALT) level of 70 iu/l and hypokalaemia (serum potassium, 3.1 mmol/l). She was once again rehydrated with normal saline and potassium chloride (40 mmol/l in each 1 l bag) and given domperidone, 60 mg per rectum three times daily, cyclizine, 50 mg intravenously three times daily and oral metoclopramide. Enoxaparin (40 mg) was given daily for thromboprophylaxis. This time she was maintained on intravenous fluids and parenteral anitemetics for 1 week. After 1 week, she was still vomiting up to three times daily and was unable to drink enough to avoid intravenous fluids. She was noted to be very depressed by her husband and the nurses caring for her and was requesting a termination of pregnancy.

The decision was made to undertake a trial of corticosteroid therapy. This was begun as hydrocortisone, 100 mg intravenously twice daily. After the first two doses, Ms F was able to tolerate oral fluids and the intravenous fluids and antiemetics were discontinued. Therapy was changed to prednisolone, 20 mg oral twice daily and she was discharged. On review in clinic 1 week later, she had had no further vomiting or nausea but still complained of "spitting". Serum electrolytes were normal, repeat liver function tests showed a normal ALT level and a repeat thyroid function test showed resolving biochemical thyrotoxicosis, with a free T$_4$ level just above the normal range. The prednisolone dose was decreased to 15 mg twice daily.

The dose was gradually weaned over the next month to 10 mg twice daily. Ptyalism had resolved by 19 weeks' gestation. An anomaly scan of the baby was normal. Several times over the next 2 months she attempted decreasing the steroid dose but would not tolerate doses below 20 mg/day. If she reduced the dose to 15 mg/day, the vomiting returned. She was thus maintained on a dose of 20 mg/day. A glucose tolerance test at 28 weeks' gestation was normal. At 30 weeks' gestation, the prednisolone dose was successfully reduced to 15 mg/day and thereafter reduced by 5 mg every 2 weeks, such that she was weaned off steroids by 36 weeks' gestation.

At 39 weeks' gestation, she presented in spontaneous labour having ruptures her membranes. She vaginally delivered a healthy female infant weighing 6 lbs 3 ozs. Postnatally, she was counselled regarding the likely recurrence of hyperemesis in future pregnancies and a plan was made to use corticosteroids at the first admission for HG.

Discussion

This was a case of severe HG causing associated abnormal liver and thyroid function. In her first pregnancy, symptoms had lasted until the third trimester and, therefore, it was likely that this would happen in any future pregnancy.

Nausea and vomiting occur commonly in pregnancy, usually between the 6th and 16th week. In 20% of cases, it persists into the second and third trimesters. Management involves reassurance, small, frequent high-carbohydrate food and avoidance of large-volume drinks. Acupunture, ginger and vitamin B6 might relieve symptoms. Other causes of vomiting in pregnancy include the following:

Ear, nose and throat diseases, for example, labyrinthitis or Meniere's disease.
Acute fatty liver of pregnancy (AFLP; in the third trimester).
HELLP syndrome.
Gastrointestinal causes, for example, cholecystitis, pancreatitis, peptic ulceration and, rarely, gastric cancer.
Metabolic/endocrine, for example, hypercalcaemia, Addison's disease and hyperparathyroidism.
Drugs, for example, opioids, iron therapy and antibiotics.
Psychological, for example, eating disorders.

If abdominal pain and tenderness is a marked feature, consideration should be given to further investigation with endoscopy.

HG is defined as vomiting occurring before the 20th week of pregnancy that is sufficient to cause dehydration, acidosis and a minimum weight loss of 5%. Some definitions include the inability to maintain the fluid and electrolyte balance without hospital admission. It occurs in about 0.5–1.5% of pregnancies and remains the third most common cause for admission to hospital during pregnancy. Before the introduction of intravenous fluids, mortality from HG was 159 deaths/1 million pregnancies. Complications of HG include Wernicke's encephalopathy, central pontine myelinosis and peripheral neuropathy. Pneumomediastinum and oesophageal rupture secondary to the mechanical forces of vomiting have been described.

Meta-analysis of the available data showed a small reduction in the risk of spontaneous miscarriage, stillbirth and preterm delivery in women who experience HG. However, when HG is severe and associated with maternal weight loss and repeated hospital admissions, there is a slight increase in the incidence of IUGR. There is no known increase in rate of congenital defects in vomiting pregnancies compared with nonvomiting pregnancies.

The aetiology of HG remains elusive. It is believed that the genetic variation in incidence is related to the presence of specific isoforms of human chorionic gonadotrophin (HCG) that cause HG [19]. Elevated levels of oestrogen and progesterone have also been implicated. Although high levels of oestrogen do cause slower intestinal transit times, there are no studies showing a relationship between severity of HG and oestrogen levels. Prospective cohort studies have not shown any consistent relationship between progesterone levels and HG.

Thyroid hormone values deviate from the normal range in early pregnancy, leading to gestational transient thyrotoxicosis [20]. Although evidence supports a relationship between HCG and gestational transient thyrotoxicosis, the exact role of this in HG is obscure. Overactivity of the adrenal cortex is also associated with HG, but it is uncertain whether it has a role in its pathogenesis. *Helicobacter pylori* infection was found in a significant number of patients with HG in 11 prospective, case-controlled studies [21]. Liver function abnormalities have been reported in about 67% of women with HG. Elevations of aspartate aminotransferase (AST) or ALT levels can be very dramatic, but return to normal with the cessation of vomiting and the end of starvation.

Clinical assessment should include measurement of the pulse, lying and standing blood pressures, urinalysis and weight, in addition to a complete examination to exclude other causes of vomiting, particularly infection. Further investigations should include urea and electrolytes, liver function tests, thyroid function tests, and serum phosphate, magnesium and calcium levels. A full blood count, midstream urine sample and blood glucose level should also be determined.

Management of HG involves rehydration with intravenous fluids, replacement of electrolytes, vitamins, antiemetics and cessation of oral nutrition and fluids. Fluid replacement can be with either sodium chloride (plus potassium, 20 mmol or 40 mmol) or Hartmann's solution. Protracted vomiting is associated with Mallory-Weiss oesophageal tears, Mendelson's syndrome and jaundice. The neurological disturbances are a result of vitamin B1 deficiency. It is imperative that thiamine hydrochloride (25–50 mg orally three times daily or as Pabrinex intravenous weekly supplements) is prescribed in these cases, to avoid Wernicke's encephalopathy and Korsakov's psychosis.

Antiemetic therapy is a mainstay of treatment, although no antiemetic treatment is specifically licensed for use in pregnancy. Pyridoxine hydrochloride (vitamin B6) and ginger have been shown to relieve symptoms in severe HG.

Dopamine receptor antagonists can be used, including the following: metoclopramide, domperidone, and phenothiazines. These drugs are safe but can cause extrapyramidal side effects. Other antiemetics that can be used include the following: cyclizine, prochlorperazine, and chlorpromazine.

Ondansetron, a potent and highly selective type 3 serotonin (5-hydroxytryptamine; 5-HT)receptor (5-HT$_3$) antagonist can be used if all other antiemetics have failed. The safety of this drug has not been sufficiently evaluated in large-scale trials. If management has been optimal and there is no improvement, consideration might be given to starting steroids (prednisolone, 20 mg twice daily or hydrocortisone, 100 mg intravenously twice daily) [22,23]. The response is usually dramatic, but if there is no response, steroids should be discontinued after 2–3 days. For those who respond to steroids, it is important to continue the therapy after discharge and wean the dose slowly. Usually, steroids will need to be continued in reduced doses until such time as nausea and vomiting have abated. With prolonged use of steroids in pregnancy, it is important to monitor blood glucose levels.

Parenteral nutrition is only recommended if there is maternal protein-calorie malnutrition and all other therapy has failed. Total parenteral nutrition (TPN) is safe, with expert advice and monitoring of maternal levels of nutrition. The fetus must be monitored with serial growth scans, and there must be facilities to accommodate preterm delivery available.

HG can be mild or severe, but most cases improve with optimal management and termination is rarely required for medical reasons. Early treatment of a recurrence is advised.

5.7 POSTPARTUM CEREBRAL HAEMORRHAGE

Ms G was a 34 year old para 2 + 5 with pre-existing renal disease and hypertension who presented 7 days after a normal vaginal delivery with sudden onset of right-sided weakness and loss of speech.

Her obstetric history was that of five miscarriages at <12 weeks' gestation. Her sixth pregnancy was complicated by severe pre-eclampsia, requiring induction at 29 weeks' gestation. She had a normal delivery of a live infant weighing 1.1 kg. Following this pregnancy, she was diagnosed with essential hypertension requiring medication. She had a renal biopsy 3 years later to investigate renal impairment and was diagnosed with Alport syndrome.

In the index pregnancy, her hypertension was controlled with methyldopa, 750 mg three times daily. Aspirin was commenced to reduce her significant risk of recurrent pre-eclampsia because of her pre-existing renal disease and hypertension, and history of previous early onset pre-eclampsia. A thrombophilia screen was negative. Renal function remained stable with serum creatinine ranging between 107–132 μmol/l. She had pre-existing significant protein-uria of 2.08 g/24 hours at the beginning of pregnancy, which dropped to 1.24 g/24 hours towards the end of the pregnancy. Serial scans confirmed normal fetal growth. There was no evidence, clinically or from blood parameters, of superimposed pre-eclampsia. She went into premature labour at 35 weeks' gestation, with a vaginal delivery of a live infant who had a birth weight of 2.2 kg. After delivery, methyldopa was converted to atenolol, 50 mg/day and her blood pressure remained stable. She was discharged home 2 days postpartum. The last blood pressure recording before discharge was 138/86 mmHg.

She was re-admitted on day 7 postpartum, having had sudden onset of headache, vomiting, one witnessed seizure, right-sided weakness and loss of speech. She had been taking atenolol, 50 mg/day for hypertension. Findings on examination were as follows: blood pressure, 182/91 mmHg; heart rate, 60 bpm; sinus rhythm; and urinalysis showed 4+ proteinuria. Neurological assessment revealed a dense right-sided hemiplegia with receptive and expressive dysphasia and a Glasgow coma scale of 11/15. Abnormal parameters on her blood results were as follows: ALT, 70 iu/l; and serum creatinine, 145 μmol/l. An urgent CT scan of the brain, with contrast, showed features suggestive of intracerebral haemorrhage in the left frontal lobe, with evidence of cerebral oedema.

She was transferred to a neurosurgical unit, where the haematoma was evacuated. This was followed by a multidisciplinary package of care on the stroke unit, involving the stroke physician, physiotherapist, speech and language therapist and clinical psychologist. She made steady progress and was able to verbalize, saying a few words and responding appropriately to commands, within 5 days of the event. Her right leg regained power, but the right arm remained flaccid. Initially, with some assistance, she was able to sit out of bed, started mobilizing by day 10 and was able to walk without supervision by day 15. During her admission, her baby was cared for at home by her mother.

She was discharged home 1 month after the event and was able to communicate well, although slowly. She had residual right-hand weakness. Power scores were 2–3 out of 5 in her right arm and 4 out of 5 in her right leg. Her hypertension was well controlled with indapamide and nifedipine. Follow-up arrangements were made with the community physiotherapist, speech and language therapist and the stroke clinic.

At her 1-year follow-up review in the stroke clinic, she had regained normal power in her right upper and lower limbs and her speech was back to normal. She had one episode of seizures and was commenced on cabamazepine. Her hypertension was well controlled with lisinopril, and simvastatin was added. She had an intrauterine contraceptive device for contraception.

Discussion

Cerebrovascular disorders are uncommon and feared complications of pregnancy. Collectively, they contributed to 15% of indirect maternal deaths in the latest confidential enquiry into maternal deaths survey. Most cases occur in the first week after delivery [24]. As highlighted in this case, there could be diagnostic confusion with eclampsia, because of the common presentation of seizures, hypertension and visual disturbance. Although Ms G had significant proteinuria at presentation, this was because of previously diagnosed underlying renal disease. Her mildly raised liver enzymes were probably a normal physiological change in the puerperium. The seizure in this case was secondary to the intracerebral bleed.

The association of pregnancy-related hypertension with stroke during pregnancy and the puerperium is consistent in many studies and with the known pathophysiology of cerebrovascular complications of hypertension.

Blood pressure at discharge after delivery is not expected to be predictive of the development of postpartum stroke. Therefore, a longer period of closer monitoring of blood pressure as an in-patient after delivery is unlikely to reduce the risk of postpartum stroke. The finding of raised blood pressure after an intracerebral bleed is related to the phenomenon of hypertension in response to seizures and central neurological insult with resulting failure of cerebral autoregulation. Hypertension is thus a result and not a cause of most cerebrovascular events.

Prompt neuroimaging studies, in addition to an elevated level of suspicion and neurological consultation, as clearly demonstrated in this case, are the key to diagnosis and an optimal prognosis. CT is usually the first imaging study performed because of its ready availability. However, an initial negative result of the CT study and the presence of a highly suggestive clinical history and physical findings suggest the need for additional studies, such as magnetic resonance imaging (MRI) and cerebral angiography, to confirm the appropriate diagnosis.

The morbidity and mortality associated with intracranial haemorrhage is high, with a risk of neurological or cardiovascular *sequelae* in survivors and a need for close medical surveillance. Ms G made a complete recovery from her hemiplegia but was left with seizures. Patients who have had stroke in the past can be reassured that they are unlikely to have a recurrence in pregnancy, unless they have an obvious risk factor, such as APS or hypertension. The combined oral contraceptive pill should be avoided because it carries a significant risk of recurrence of stroke. Ms G was advised to seek prepregnancy counselling before embarking on another pregnancy.

5.8 HYPOKALAEMIA

Mrs H was a 31 year old primigravida who presented at 26 weeks' gestation with extreme lethargy such that she was virtually bed bound. She had a diagnosis of Sjogren's syndrome and was anti-Ro and anti-La positive. Her pregnancy had been complicated by recurrent admissions for HG, and on each occasion she was noted to be hypokalaemic (serum potassium, 2.4–3.1 mmol/l), which improved with appropriate rehydration with normal saline and potassium chloride. However, at this admission she denied nausea or vomiting, which had improved markedly since 20 weeks' gestation.

Investigations revealed a serum potassium level of 2.9 mmol/l and serum bicarbonate of 14 mmol/l. Retrospective review of biochemistry results during the previous admissions showed that on each admission she had been acidotic, with serum bicarbonate levels as low as 10 mmol/l. Because persistent vomiting in HG usually causes a hypochloraemic alkalosis (related to the loss of hydrochloric acid from the stomach), alternative causes for the hypokalaemia were considered. Because of the association of Sjogren's syndrome with distal type 1 renal tubular acidosis (RTA), this was felt to be the most likely diagnosis. Urinary pH was 9 when serum bicarbonate was 15 mmol/l. This was highly suggestive of RTA.

Treatment was commenced with oral sodium bicarbonate, 1.8 g three times daily and oral potassium citrate, 10 ml (28 mmol/l/10 ml) three times daily. Within 1 week, she had normal energy levels and felt enormously better. Within 2 weeks, her serum bicarbonate and potassium levels were normal and potassium supplementation was discontinued.

Mrs H was delivered by emergency Caesarean section for fetal distress at 38 weeks' gestation; the birth weight of her infant was 3.1 kg. Postpartum, the dose of bicarbonate was reduced to 1.2 g three times daily. She was referred to a nephrologist for further management postpartum.

Discussion

Hypokalaemia occurs in up to 20% of hospitalized patients but is only clinically apparent in 5%. No pregnancy-specific incidence has been reported. Hypokalaemia is a biochemical finding and is not a diagnosis in itself. It is almost always secondary to an underlying problem.

Hypokalaemia is frequently asymptomatic. Severe hypokalaemia (serum potassium, <2.5 mmol/l) can cause muscle weakness and fatigue. It rarely causes arrhythmia in patients without cardiac disease.

Despite the 50% increase in plasma volume and associated haemo-dilution of pregnancy, the concentration of plasma electrolytes remains unchanged compared with the nonpregnant state. The range of normal serum potassium is 3.5–5.5 mmol/l. This phenomenon is probably because of decreased excretion in pregnancy and net gain from gastric absorption. In rat studies, fluctuations in maternal serum potassium levels did not seem to have a deleterious effect on fetal potassium levels.

Hypokalaemia has many causes. Acute hypokalaemia is most commonly due to severe vomiting and/or diarrhoea. Chronic hypokalaemia is most commonly due to diuretic use and hyperaldosteronism. A logical review of possible causes of potassium loss should facilitate the correct diagnosis:

Renal losses:
- RTA
- Hyperaldosteronism
- Hypomagnesaemia
- Leukaemia

Gastrointestinal losses:
- Vomiting or nasogastric suctioning
- Diarrhoea
- Enemas/laxatives
- Ileal loop

Drugs:
- Diuretics (except potassium-sparing diuretics)
- Beta-adrenoceptor agonists
- Steroids
- Aminophyllins
- Aminoglycosides

Transcellular shifts:
- Insulin
- Alkalosis

Reduced intake:
- Dietary deficiency, including malnutrition
- Parenteral nutrition
- Intravenous fluids lacking potassium

The following are pregnancy-specific/related causes:

HG
Tocolysis with intravenous sympathomimetics, such as salbutamol [25].
Oral glucose load screening for gestational diabetes [26].
Abnormal cravings in pregnancy (pica), such as cravings for cola or clay, and caffeine abuse in pregnancy [27,28,29].

A thorough search for the aetiology of hypokalaemia is required. It will generally resolve with the treatment of its primary cause. Supportive replacement therapy is, however, indicated in 5% of patients, where the potassium level is <3 mmol/l. Oral therapy is usually sufficient. However, intravenous therapy might be indicated if symptoms are severe, cardiac arrhythmias are present and oral intake is not possible (vomiting or diarrhoea). Potassium supplementation is safe in pregnancy. When hypokalaemia is refractory to treatment, hypomagnesaemia should be suspected and corrected concurrently.

RTA is systemic acidosis due to the inability of the renal tubules to maintain the acid–base balance. Type 4 RTA is the commonest form, but it is associated with hyperkalaemia. RTA types 1 and 2 are associated with hypokalaemia. Type 2 (proximal) RTA is very rare. Type 1 (distal) RTA is usually secondary to systemic conditions such as diabetic ketoacidosis, liver disease, sickle cell anaemia and autoimmune conditions, including Sjogren's syndrome (as present in Mrs H), thyrotoxicosis and systemic lupus erythematosus (SLE). It can be sporadic, in which case it is usually an autosomal dominant familial condition. Characteristically, there is failure to acidify the urine despite systemic acidosis. It is characterized by episodes of weakness and paralysis and is accompanied by hypokalaemia, acidosis and hypocalcaemia. Diagnosis is usually made following an acid-load test, during which the patient takes an oral solution of ammonium chloride; if the urine fails to acidify but the bicarbonate level falls, this is diagnostic of RTA. Treatment is usually supportive with potassium, bicarbonate and calcium supplementation during episodes.

During pregnancy, symptoms such as fatigue and lethargy can mimic muscular weakness and make the diagnosis even harder to reach. The ammonium load test is contraindicated in pregnancy because acidosis can cause fetal distress. Untreated RTA can cause severe weakness affecting labour and maternal well-being. Chronic acidosis affects fetal bone growth, causing IUGR, and can cause cardiotocographic changes. Potassium, bicarbonate and calcium supplementation is safe in pregnancy. The potassium and bicarbonate requirements are sevenfold and fourfold higher, respectively, in pregnancy than outside pregnancy.

In a review by Hardadottir et al. [30], RTA cases were associated with IUGR, preterm labour and Caesarean section. Most cases of RTA were secondary. It seems prudent to follow RTA pregnancies with serial fetal growth scans and institute intrapartum cardiotocographic monitoring. Neonatal admissions were common in the above mentioned series, and therefore paediatric colleagues should be involved before delivery. If tocolysis is required, it is best to avoid beta-sympathomimetics because they induce hyperglycaemia and hypokalaemia.

In labour, attention should be paid to avoid potential precipitating factors, including mental and physical stress, cold and carbohydrate loads. Adequate analgesia should be administered, and an early epidural might be ideal. Serum potassium should be monitored and replaced as necessary, usually intravenously. The second stage of labour can be shortened with assisted delivery if maternal exhaustion or fetal distress supervenes. Glucose infusions should be avoided because they can precipitate further hypokalaemia.

In the first 2 weeks of the puerperium, potassium, bicarbonate and calcium supplementation usually decreases rapidly towards prepregnancy doses. If the diagnosis has not been confirmed, the ammonium load test can be completed postnatally.

5.9 HEPATITIS A

Mrs J, a 28 year old nulliparous woman at 34 weeks' gestation, was admitted with a history of worsening malaise, diarrhoea, nausea and vomiting, and generalized itching. There was associated dark urine, but no paleness of stools. Her pregnancy had being uneventful apart from intermittent diarrhoea, presumed to be secondary to her history of irritable bowel syndrome and managed with loperamide. Her booking bloods at the beginning of the pregnancy, were negative for human immunodeficiency virus (HIV) and hepatitis B. She was from South Africa and had been a resident in the UK for 3 years. She worked as a secondary school teacher. There was no history of recent travel, or use of herbal remedies or hepatotoxic drugs.

On examination, she was afebrile and jaundiced, with normal blood pressure and without proteinuria on urine dipstick assessment and signs of chronic liver disease apart from telangectasia over the upper chest and abdomen, which was associated with pregnancy. Abdominal examination revealed no organomegaly and her fundal height was consistent with gestational age. Fetal movements were normal and the cardiotocograph (CTG) was reactive. Blood tests revealed a normal full blood count, with Hb concentration of 12.5 g/dl, white blood cell count of 9.6×10^9 cells/l and platelet count of 198×10^9 platelets/l. Her renal function and random blood glucose were normal, but her liver function was de-ranged (bilirubin, 98 μmol/l; ALT, 769 iu/l; alkaline phosphatase (AlkP), 185 iu/l; gamma-GT, 47 iu/l; and serum albumin, 24 g/l). Her coagulation was normal.

She was transferred into a side room and barrier-nursed, with institution of mainly supportive management, in addition to antihistamines and vitamin K. Upper abdominal ultrasound revealed a normal liver, gallbladder and spleen. Cultures of blood, urine and sputum were negative.

Over the next 2 days, she gradually improved clinically, in addition to biochemically (Table 3). Serum titres for hepatitis A revealed a raised immunoglobulin (Ig) M consistent with acute hepatitis A infection. Titres for hepatitis B and C were negative. Antimitochondrial and anti-smooth muscle antibodies were negative. She was discharged home after 1 week because she continued to improve.

She went into premature labour at 36 weeks' gestation and had a normal vaginal delivery of a male infant, weighing 2.8 kg. By 2 weeks post delivery, her liver function had normalized.

Discussion

Liver disease in pregnancy can be subdivided into three types:

1. Liver disease peculiar to pregnancy, such as AFLP, obstetric cholestasis, HG and pre-eclampsia.

2. Intercurrent liver disease affecting pregnant women, such as viral hepatitis and gall bladder disease.
3. The effect of pregnancy on underlying liver disease, such as chronic hepatitis or cirrhosis.

Clearly, the last category was not considered as a differential diagnosis in this case because there was no previous history of liver disease. As a symptom of liver disease, jaundice occurs in 1:1500 pregnancies: 40% of cases result from viral hepatitis, 20% of cases are secondary to intrahepatic cholestasis, and < 6% of cases result from common biliary duct obstruction and gallstones. A normal gall bladder scan excluded the latter in this patient.

Pruritus can occur in a broad spectrum of liver disease and its presence does not necessarily help in reaching the correct diagnosis. Although pruritus classically occurs in conditions associated with intrahepatic cholestasis, such as primary biliary cirrhosis and obstetric cholestasis, drug hepatotoxicity, viral hepatitis, AFLP and even pre-eclampsia are sometimes associated with itching. The absence of antimitochondrial antibodies and lack of a positive history of drug ingestion excluded primary biliary cirrhosis (PBC) and drug-induced causes in Mrs J.

The length of gestation at presentation is important in considering possible diagnoses because, unlike viral hepatitis, which can occur at anytime, liver disease specifically associated with pregnancy occurs at characteristic times. In the third trimester, HELLP syndrome, AFLP, obstetric cholestasis and pre-eclampsia (PET) should be considered.

The pattern of serum liver enzyme abnormalities cannot be relied on to make a diagnosis. Classically, in intrahepatic liver disease, transaminases tend to be high, with only a small increase in alkaline phosphatase; in extrahepatic obstruction, alkaline phosphatase is high and transaminases are relatively lower. In Mrs J, the pattern was consistent with the picture in viral hepatitis, drug-induced hepatotoxicity, obstetric cholestasis, AFLP, HELLP syndrome and PET. The absence of thrombocytopenia, which is one of the hallmarks of HELLP syndrome, and impaired liver function (coagulation and glucose were both normal), which is a prominent feature of AFLP, made these two conditions unlikely. There is a tendency in pregnancy to assume that pruritus is always due to obstetric cholestasis: it was vital in this case that the viral titres were obtained quickly, because this enabled the correct diagnosis to be made.

Viral hepatitis is mostly due to hepatitis A, B, C, D or E, Epstein-Barr virus, or cytomegalovirus. Pregnant women are not more susceptible to hepatitis, and the incidence in epidemics is usually

TABLE 5.3. Results of investigations during illness and at follow-up

Gestation, weeks + days	34 + 4	34 + 5	34 + 6	35 + 2	35 + 5	36 + 1	36 + 4	2 weeks postdelivery
Hb, g/dl	12.5	13.5	12.1	12.7	13.8	13.8	13.8	14.8
WBC, × 10⁹/l	9.6	9.9	9.3	8.1	12.8	11.6	10.5	10.2
Platelet count, × 10⁹ platelets/l	198	222	269	284	354	397	457	343
Creatinine, µmol/l		57	63	56				
K, mmol/l			3.6					
Uric acid, mmol/l		0.20	0.25					
Bilirubin, µmol/l	98	108	62	62	31	24	14	13
Total protein, g/l	54		50	54	61	69		70
Albumin, g/l	24	25	22	25	27	27	32	42
ALT, iu/l	769	711	445	439	237	534	366	51
Alkaline phosphatase, iu/l	185	200	178	190	219	176	157	85
gamma-GT, iu/l		47	48	65	56	53	48	21

ALT - alanine transaminase; GT - gamma-glutamyl transpeptidase; Hb - haemoglobin; K - potassium; WBC - white blood cells.

the same in pregnant and nonpregnant women. However, hepatitis E is more aggressive in pregnancy, with a maternal mortality rate of up to 50% [31].

Acute hepatitis A in pregnancy is a systemic, short-term viral illness, with general symptoms of malaise and jaundice. It is the most common cause of jaundice in pregnancy [32]. The virus belongs to the picornaviridae RNA family. Transmission is through the faeco-oral route, and it is endemic in countries with poor sanitation. The incubation period is generally 15–50 days. It multiplies in the intestine and invades the blood, liver and saliva before any clinical manifestation of the disease appears. It is highly contagious, with maximal viral shedding occurring in the 1–2 week period before the onset of symptoms and lasting 3 weeks. The virus disappears soon after the peak of serum transaminases is reached, at which time the immune response and hepatocellular repair start. The risk of transmission diminishes following the onset of symptoms and is minimal in the week after the onset of jaundice.

Hepatitis A is not debilitating, even in the presence of jaundice. Jaundice lasts 7–10 days and the whole illness lasts about 4 weeks. Typically, all clinical forms, with the exception of the rare, lethal, fulminant type, resolve with complete liver regeneration, and without chronicity or long-term carrier state. Serum IgM antibodies are present during the acute phase and disappear within 3 months. Serum IgG antibodies develop after the acute illness and persist for life, representing immunity. Serum transaminases rise with acute illness and return to normal with recovery; they seldom are higher than 1000 iu/l. There is no correlation between their level and prognosis.

Maternal–fetal transmission is rare but could result if the mother has hepatitis at or around the time of delivery. In such cases, the baby should be given Ig at birth. It is recommended that pregnant women who are exposed to hepatitis A are given Ig prophylaxis, because it reduces the risk of infection. Ig must be given within 2 weeks of exposure but should be given as soon as possible.

Hepatitis A vaccination (inactivated noninfectious hepatitis A virus) is not contraindicated in pregnancy. It is recommended for some individuals working in high-risk professions, people travelling to at-risk countries and individuals with medical conditions that place them at a high risk of complications from hepatitis A. It offers good protection and is thought to be effective for 20 years.

Breastfeeding can continue without interruption if a mother has hepatitis A. If the mother becomes acutely ill or jaundiced, breastfeeding might be interrupted. The mother should practise good handwashing and other appropriate hygiene.

Acute hepatitis A is the commonest cause of viral hepatitis in pregnancy; it is usually self-limiting and nondebilitating and is associated with transient abnormal liver function, mostly with no significant implications to the pregnancy. It is vital that abnormal liver function in pregnancy is investigated fully so that the correct diagnosis is reached.

5.10 RENAL ARTERY STENOSIS

Mrs K was a 25 year old Asian woman who presented in her third pregnancy at 22 weeks' gestation with severe secondary hypertension. She was diagnosed with bilateral renal artery stenosis following a limited angiogram during her second pregnancy, when she was found to be severely hypertensive. She unfortunately miscarried her second pregnancy at 20 weeks' gestation. Her first pregnancy was a termination at 9 weeks' gestation. Following her miscarriage, she had a left renal artery angioplasty, and the right angioplasty was planned as an interval procedure. Before having the right renal artery angioplasty, she was found to be pregnant. It was felt that angioplasty during pregnancy would, on one hand, be an unwarranted radiation dose but, in contrast, would reduce the risk of severe hypertension.

She booked-in late in her third pregnancy at 22 weeks' gestation with a blood pressure of 199/125 mmHg, despite therapy with two agents, atenolol (50 mg once daily) and doxazosin (4 mg twice daily). Methyldopa (500 mg three times daily) and aspirin (75 mg once daily) were added. Booking bloods were normal, in addition to baseline renal function: urea, 3.5 mmol/l; creatinine, 65 μmol/l; uric acid, 0.31 mmol/l. Urinalysis was normal and 24-hour urine protein leak was 0.24 g/save. An obstetric scan at 22 weeks' gestation revealed bilateral uterine artery Doppler notching, with a raised resistance index.

Mrs K was closely monitored and her blood pressure remained well controlled on the above three antihypertensive agents. At 26 weeks' gestation, a growth scan revealed evidence of IUGR with reduced liquor volume and AC below the fifth centile. An umbilical artery Doppler scan showed absent end diastolic flow. Estimated fetal weight (EFW) was 669 g. She was admitted because of the scan finding and also to exclude a possible diagnosis of pre-eclampsia. Investigations for pre-eclampsia were normal and the protein leak remained nonsignificant. The risk of a poor outcome, including a high risk of intrauterine death, reduced chance of neonatal survival and significant risk of neurological impairment, was discussed. It was decided to avoid delivery at this gestation and wait for the fetus to gain more maturity. Mrs K was discharged home with a plan for weekly umbilical Doppler scans and 2-weekly growth scans.

Her blood pressure remained stable and well controlled, with no signs of superimposed pre-eclampsia. At 30 weeks' gestation, her scan revealed no fetal growth in 4 weeks, brain sparing and anhydramnios. It was felt that delivery was now necessary because the additional weeks gained had improved the fetal prognosis. She had a course of steroids and was delivered 24 hours later, at 30 weeks + 6 days, by Caesarean section with an inverted T-incision on the uterus; Apgar scores at delivery were 9 and 10 at 1 minute and 5 minutes, respectively, and the infant had a birth weight of 815 g. Postoperatively, she was converted to her prepregnancy antihypertensive medication, with good blood pressure control. The neonatal course was complicated by necrotizing enterocolitis, which required surgical intervention, with subsequent full recovery. She was referred to the renal physician for renal angioplasty.

Discussion

Renovascular hypertension is one of the potentially curable secondary causes of hypertension. It is the cause of hypertension in <5% of all patients. In women of child-bearing age, fibromuscular hyperplasia is more often the aetiology. Patients with renal artery stenosis usually present with hypertension and varying degrees of renal impairment. Narrowing of the renal artery, because of fibromuscular dysplasia, leads to reduced renal perfusion. The consequent activation of renin–angiotensin system causes hypertension (mediated by angiotensin II), hypokalaemia and hypernatraemia (which are features of secondary hyperaldosteronism). Correcting the stenosis might reverse these features and improve hypertension control.

Before her first angioplasty, Mrs K required three antihypertensive agents, which was reduced to two agents after the angioplasty. It would be expected that following angioplasty of the other renal artery a cure might be achieved, without the need for medication.

Secondary, potentially curable causes of hypertension should be sought whenever hypertension is present in young women, whether pregnant or not. This is especially true for pre-existing hypertension in pregnancy that has not been previously diagnosed. Clinical features and pointers to a diagnosis of renal artery stenosis are as follows: young hypertensive patients with no family history, resistant hypertension, >1.5 cm difference in kidney size on ultrasonography, and secondary hyperaldosteronism (low plasma potassium concentration). Clinical examination might reveal bruits over major vessels, including the abdominal aorta.

Angiography remains the standard test for diagnosis, but it is not without risks and could worsen renal function. Noninvasive techniques are beginning to replace conventional angiography. These include Doppler ultrasonography, captopril renography, spiral CT scanning and magnetic resonance angiography. The significance of lesions found by renal arteriography should be confirmed by differential renal function studies and renal venous renin activity before surgical management is undertaken. The severity of stenosis determines treatment. Hypertension caused by slight or moderate stenosis commonly responds favourably to medical management.

The concern in pregnancy, and especially in the case discussed, was the risk of the radiation dose involved with angiography. Mrs K had had a renal angiogram in her second pregnancy, which resulted in the diagnosis of renal artery stenosis, but subsequently miscarried. Although one can argue that the radiation dose involved with an angiogram would not be greater than the maximum allowed in pregnancy (~5 rad), it was felt wise to avoid angioplasty in the subsequent pregnancy because the patient perceived the angiogram as a possible causal factor for the miscarriage. It is more likely that this late miscarriage related to severe hypertension rather than radiation. By contrast, performing the second angioplasty in the third pregnancy might have led to a better outcome for the patient and her fetus. Although Mrs K's blood pressure was well controlled by antihypertensive therapy, poor fetal growth resulted from the effects of hypertension on placental perfusion, which might have been avoided if an angioplasty had been carried out in the pregnancy.

Angioplasty is the traditional revascularization procedure, and this often leads to cure in patients with fibromuscular dysplasia. Resistant hypertension secondary to fibromuscular dysplasia has been the primary indication cited for dilatation of the renal artery. Although a modest improvement in blood pressure or reduction in antihypertensive drug requirement might be the goal of revascularization, renal protection could emerge as the more important factor.

Drugs alone can control hypertension in almost 90% of patients with renal artery stenosis. Antihypertensive therapy during pregnancy might need to be adjusted. Methyldopa, labetalol, hydralazine and nifedipine are safe. Angiotensin receptor blockers and ACE inhibitors are contraindicated in pregnant women and in renal artery stenosis. It is important to note that lowering blood pressure might decrease uteroplacental perfusion and impair fetal growth.

Renal artery stenosis is an uncommon secondary cause of hypertension in pregnancy, which can be associated with poorly controlled hypertension and poor fetal outcome. It can usually be managed with antihypertensive medication, but definitive treatment is revascularization with angioplasty, which should be considered in pregnancy, in the face of resistant hypertension.

5.11 THYROID CANCER

Ms L was a 34 year old nulliparous caucasian woman who presented to her GP at 11 weeks' gestation complaining of a thyroid lump, which she had noticed during the preceeding year. On examination, she was clinically euthyroid. An irregular mass was palpable in the right lobe of the thyroid, measuring 5 cm × 3 cm. There was no bruit or palpable lymphadenopathy. An ultrasound scan confirmed a solid thyroid mass, with a 9 mm lymph node at its inferio-lateral aspect. Fine-needle aspiration (FNA) of the thyroid mass was suggestive of papillary thyroid carcinoma. Biochemically she was euthyroid. She was commenced on a suppressive dose of thyroxine, 300 μg/day.

Mrs L was reviewed at a tertiary oncology centre at 12 weeks' gestation. A repeat FNA confirmed the diagnosis of papillary thyroid carcinoma, and an MRI confirmed nodal involvement. She had a total thyroidectomy with selective right-neck dissection and conservation of two parathyroid glands at 16 weeks' gestation. Histology reported complete excision of a 4 cm papillary carcinoma with follicular pattern, with extranodal extension but no extension to the capsule. Because of the constellation of adverse pathological features (i.e. the site, nodal involvement and extranodal spread), radio- iodine ablation was planned after delivery. Her pregnancy progressed well, with a satisfactory growth scan at 32 weeks' gestation. Her thyroid function was regularly monitored, with TSH level moderately suppressed to a low-to-middle range of normal (0.5–2.8 mu/1). Her free T_4 level was 14 pmol/l on a dose of 200 μg of thyroxine. Her corrected calcium level was initially low and required calcium supplementation, which was discontinued after the calcium level normalized.

Mrs L went into spontaneous labour at 39 weeks' gestation and was delivered by vacuum extraction of a live infant in good condition and with birth weight of 3.41 kg. At 6 weeks postpartum, her TSH level was significantly suppressed, at <0.1 mu/1, with a free T_4 level of 21.5 pmol/l on a dose of 200 μg of thyroxine. This dose was reduced to 150 μg. She was clinically euthyroid and was supplementing breastfeeding with bottle feeding. At 3 months postdelivery, when her T_4 had been suspended for several weeks, she had radio-iodine ablation treatment. She was advised not to conceive within the next 6–12 months and to avoid close contact with her baby for 3–4 weeks.

Discussion

Half of all thyroid cancers occur in women of child-bearing age, but presentation in pregnancy is rare, occurring in approximately 1 in 10,000 pregnancies. The most common complaint is that of a thyroid nodule, but these occur in up to 5% of women of child-bearing age, and only a small proportion are malignant. Overall, most authorities believe that pregnancy neither stimulates the growth of thyroid cancer nor worsens the prognosis [33].

If thyroid cancer is diagnosed before the mid-trimester, surgical intervention can be performed with normal surgical management, as in the case described above. Recent data suggest that the risk of fetal loss related to surgery is minimal. When the diagnosis is reached during late pregnancy, resection after delivery is the option of choice, with surgery being performed once the pregnancy-associated vascularity is judged to have resolved. In women whose FNA suggests a well-differentiated tumour, some studies have shown no difference in the outcome between those patients that had early surgery and those patients who had surgery delayed. There is no indication for termination of pregnancy, although if the tumour is felt to be aggressive or disseminated, early delivery might be appropriate, in which case the balance of risks of fetal and maternal well-being must be carefully assessed [34].

In this case, radio-iodine ablation was indicated postdelivery. T_4 must be stopped 4 weeks before treatment to enable the TSH level to rise, which facilitates uptake of iodine into the residual thyroid tissue. Pregnancy should be delayed usually for at least 12 months after radio-iodine treatment, because it has a long half-life and is associated with an increased risk of miscarriage and congenital abnormality if conception occurs sooner. In addition, this time period enables appropriate suppression of TSH to be achieved; if there is an early recurrence, management is easier. Clearly, radio-iodine should not be given in pregnancy: inadvertent use in the early second trimester causes fetal thyroid destruction and subsequent hypothyroidism [35].

The mammary gland binds iodide avidly, especially during lactation, so if radio-iodine treatment is required, breastfeeding should be stopped and contact with the baby reduced to limit the radiation to the child to the lowest levels: the length of time is determined by the dose of radioactive iodine required, but is often around 3 weeks [36].

The prognosis of most thyroid cancers is excellent. Many women are maintained on a suppressive dose of thyroxine, aiming for an undetectable TSH level, and so minimizing the risk of stimulation of any residual thyroid tumour. Subsequent pregnancies do not alter the risk of disease recurrence, but for women on a suppressive dose of T_4, thyroid function should be monitored and the dose adjusted as indicated.

5.12 ABDOMINAL PAIN

Ms M was a 24 year old para 1 + 1 who presented to the antenatal day unit at 30 + 2 weeks' gestation with a history of a fall on a wet surface that caused some bruising on the left leg and left side of the abdomen. Her examination was normal and no uterine contractions, vaginal discharge or bleeding were noted. A CTG was normal, and after being given anti-D for a rhesus-negative blood type, she was discharged.

Her past obstetric history was of one miscarriage at 9 weeks' gestation and one Caesarean section at 41 weeks' gestation (delivering a 2.5 kg baby) because of suspected fetal distress after prostaglandin administration for induction of labour. Her past medical history included mild asthma, for which she was using regular salbutamol and beclomethasone inhalers.

At 31 + 1 weeks' gestation, Ms M was admitted with continuing abdominal pain and decreased fetal movements. The abdominal pain was in the left iliac fossa, constant in nature and made worse by movement. No cause for the abdominal pain could be found and fetal assessment, with both CTG and umbilical artery Doppler scanning, was normal. Fetal movements returned to normal the day after admission. Ms M was reviewed at 31 + 6 weeks' gestation and had continuing left iliac fossa pain, which radiated to her back and was constant in nature, but worse on movement. While in the day unit waiting for the results of repeat blood tests, she noticed sudden-onset epigastric pain, which was associated with shortness of breath, a nonproductive cough and inspiratory chest pain. On examination, her heart rate was 100 bpm, her respiratory rate was 28 per minute, her temperature was normal and her blood pressure was 117/65 mmHg. The jugular venous pressure (JVP) was not raised, the chest was clear on auscultation and heart sounds were normal. Neither calf was tender. Her oxygen saturation on air was 94%. After 1 hour, she started complaining of dizziness at rest.

Further urgent investigations included a 12-lead ECG, which showed a sinus tachycardia, a full blood count, which showed polymorphonuclear leukocytosis, liver function tests, which were normal, and measurement of serum amylase and C-reactive protein. Arterial blood gases showed a pH of 7.431, pCO_2 of 3.59 kPa and a pO_2 of 9.1 kPa (hypoxaemia). A chest X-ray was normal.

Pulmonary thromboembolism was felt to be the most likely diagnosis and therapy was commenced with a therapeutic dose of enoxaparin (1 mg/kg body weight/twice daily). The following day, a (V/Q) lung scan confirmed bilateral ventilation perfusion mismatches consistent with pulmonary emboli. Her leg vein Doppler scans showed extensive thrombus in the left iliac vein.

Anticoagulation was continued until 39 + 2 weeks' gestation, when Ms M went into spontaneous labour. Because a dose of 80 mg of enoxaparin had been given 6 hours before the request for epidural analgesia, this was declined. Pain relief was achieved with patient-controlled intravenous opiate analgesia and Ms M had a spontaneous vaginal delivery of a 2.9 kg baby boy. The estimated blood loss was 300 ml. Following delivery and 26 hours after her last dose of enoxaparin, anticoagulation was restarted with enoxaparin, 120 mg once daily (1.5 mg/kg body weight once daily). Warfarin was commenced at a dose of 7 mg on day 3, and by day 6, the international normalized ration (INR) was 2.3 and the enoxaparin was discontinued. Warfarin was continued for a further 3 months postpartum. A thrombophilia screen after the discontinuation of warfarin showed that Ms M was heterozygous for factor V Leiden.

Discussion

Ms M had several risk factors for venous thromboembolism. She was pregnant and had recently sustained a minor injury that had left her relatively immobile. Her mother had suffered a deep vein thrombosis (DVT) aged 42 years.

Included in the differential diagnosis of the epigastric and pleuritic pain should be an atypical acute asthmatic episode, pneumonia, pneumothorax, ischaemic/cardiac causes, aortic dissection, cholecystitis, pancreatitis and gastro-oesophageal reflux. The presence of hypoxia made pulmonary embolism a likely diagnosis.

Arterial blood gases in pulmonary embolism might show hypoxaemia, as in Ms M, with or without hypocapnia caused by hyperventilation to compensate for the loss of pulmonary function. In a small pulmonary embolism hyperventilation causing respiratory alkalosis might be the first change in arterial blood gases. Using pulse oximetry, a drop in oxygen saturation after exercise (such as walking up and down a flight of stairs) is a useful screening test if the oxygen saturation at rest is normal. In normal pregnancy, there is relative hypocapnia because of the increased respiratory work of pregnancy, such that the normal pCO$_2$ is 3.5–4.5 kPa, approximately 1 kPa lower than outside pregnancy.

D-dimer measurement in pregnancy is not useful. In nonpregnant women they are thought to be fairly sensitive, but nonspecific, for thrombosis and therefore are helpful, if negative, to exclude diagnosis of thrombosis. In the pregnant woman, there is a physiological rise in D-dimers, but normal ranges for pregnancy have not been fully established, such that the false-positive rate is high [37].

In retrospect, it is likely that the left iliac fossa pain was due to iliac vein thrombosis, which then dislodged to cause the pulmonary embolism. Iliac vein thrombosis is more common on the left-hand side in pregnancy because the inferior vena cava runs on the right-hand side of the aorta and therefore the left iliac vein is more likely to be compressed by the right iliac artery. DVT in pregnancy is eight to nine times more common on the left than the right [38,39].

Alternative to awaiting spontaneous labour would have been induction of labour or elective repeat Caesarean section. Both these strategies would have allowed planned temporary interruption of LMWH to permit regional analgesia or anaesthesia, but the latter would have increased the risk of thrombosis compared with vaginal delivery. However, Ms M was keen for a vaginal birth after Caesarean section (VBAC) and induction of labour was not felt to be desirable because of the previous Caesarean section, and because it might have introduced extended bed rest and dehydration. It is important that women receiving therapeutic LMWH are seen and counselled by an obstetric anaesthetist before delivery so that the issues surrounding options for analgesia and anaesthesia can be discussed before delivery.

5.13 MITRAL STENOSIS

Ms N was a 26 year old primiparous woman from East Africa who booked-in at her local hospital in the sixth week of her pregnancy. She was known to have "mild mitral stenosis" from an echocardiogram she had following an earlier miscarriage. She had previously been investigated, but the results of those investigations were not known. She had mild asthma and used a salbutamol inhaler for this on an "as required" basis. She was also a smoker.

Ms N presented locally at 24 weeks' gestation with possible haemoptysis. The differential diagnosis was haematemesis and gastroscopy was carried out, in addition to a V/Q scan and sputum microscopy and culture, to exclude tuberculosis. The gastroscopy, under antibiotic cover, revealed a Mallory-Weiss tear and she was therefore prescribed raniti-dine. An echocardiogram repeated at this time confirmed "mild mitral stenosis" and at this time Ms N was asymptomatic. At 26 weeks'gesta-tion, she was becoming breathless on climbing stairs, but could still walk well on the flat. There was no orthopnoea. An anaesthetic opinion was arranged.

At 35 weeks' gestation, Ms N was admitted through the accident and emergency department to a tertiary obstetric unit. She gave a history of 4 hours of cough, pink frothy sputum and no response to her inhaler. There was also associated pleuritic chest pain. A malar flush, typical of mitral stenosis, was also evident [40].

On examination, she had a pulse rate of 130 bpm, her blood pres-sure was 84/51 mmHg, her respiratory rate was 18 breaths per minute and she had a PEFR of 300 l/min. The JVP was elevated, and she had a mid-diastolic murmur and bibasal lung crepitations. Oxygen saturation was 97% in room air. An ECG revealed a sinus tachycardia and the chest X-ray showed consolidation at the right base. Obstetrically, all was well. She was given frusemide, 40 mg intravenously and diamorphine, 5 mg intravenously, with oxygen, by mask, at 5 l/min. The transthoracic echocardiogram showed rheu-matic mitral stenosis of moderate severity, with a dilated left atrium (5.6 cm), mitral valve area of 1.1 cm^2 and mean gradient of 8.5 mmHg (normal, 0–2), and good biventricular function. The diag-nosis was pulmonary oedema, related to mitral stenosis.

A history of 7 years of dyspnoea was then obtained through the husband; dyspnoea was worse in pregnancy, with orthopnoea and paroxysmal nocturnal dyspnoea. He also reported recent onset of haemoptysis and a much reduced exercise tolerance, i.e. five steps up a flight of stairs.

Treatment commenced with regular frusemide and diltiazem. Diltiazem was used to control the heart rate instead of a beta-blocker, because of the history of asthma. She was also commenced on LMWH prophylaxis and required potassium supplementation. Amiloride was added to frusemide for potassium conservation. Despite this therapy, she remained tachycardic. Diltiazem was, there-fore, increased and the option of balloon valvotomy was discussed, should medical therapy fail to prevent further episodes of pulmonary oedema. Ms N was placed on a 1500 ml/24 hours fluid restriction regimen as an adjunct to drug therapy.

By day 3 after admission, her heart rate had dropped below 100 bpm and she was less dyspnoeic. By day 4, there was still signif-icant difficulty maintaining the serum potassium; therefore, the amiloride dose was doubled. She was also given an infusion of 8 mM of magnesium in 100 ml of physiological saline, to help maintain her potassium level and prevent atrial fibrillation. After a few more days of diuretics in combination with fluid restriction (1500 ml/24 hours), she became asymptomatic. Induction of labour was scheduled for 38 weeks' gestation. An obstetric anaesthetic opinion was obtained and a plan was made for an elective epidural.

At 38 weeks' gestation, Ms N went into spontaneous labour. During labour, fluids were restricted to 85 ml/hour. Antibiotics were given for endocarditis prophylaxis and care was taken to avoid the lithotomy and supine positions. Labour progressed well until augmentation was necessary, with a low-volume Syntocinon infusion, at 9 cm. The morning diuretic dose was administered as usual. After pushing for 35 minutes she was delivered, with the ventouse and a right medio-lateral episiotomy. The estimated blood loss was 200 ml.

Ms N had routine postnatal care, with an appointment scheduled for valvotomy. She was advised not to conceive again before treatment of the valve. Warfarin was commenced on the third postnatal day and Ms N was discharged with sustained-release diltiazem and co-amilofruse. She was also given contraceptive advice, choosing Depo-Provera as her preferred method. She underwent balloon mitral valvuloplasty 2 months later; her postprocedure echocardiogram showed a mitral valve area of 2.2 cm².

Discussion

Globally, rheumatic heart disease is the most common cardiac disease presenting in pregnancy, with mitral stenosis the commonest lesion [41]. The most likely time for complications to present is during the late second and third trimesters, as occurred in this case and can be expected in up to 60% of all cases. Complications are usually pulmonary oedema, arrhythmias or deterioration in New York Heart Association (NYHA) functional class [41].

Ms N presented during the third trimester with pulmonary oedema, which took a long time to bring under control. The deterioration seemed to be associated with pneumonia (basal consolidation on chest X-ray) [42] and a tachycardia of 130 bpm, which resulted in elevation of left atrial pressure (as evidenced by a dilated left atrium on echocardiography) and pulmonary oedema. If the medical measures had been unsuccessful in treating her pulmonary oedema, a mitral valvotomy would have been undertaken, which would have improved cardiac function significantly for labour and delivery [41].

Therapeutic strategies include off-loading the heart by reducing both preload (volume) and afterload (peripheral resistance). Ms N immediately received emergency treatment for pulmonary oedema with diamorphine, frusemide and oxygen. With the history of haemoptysis, one of the most obvious diagnoses to exclude would be pulmonary embolus, which might have explained the tachycardia and basal consolidation. However, an urgent echocardiogram showed no evidence of acute pulmonary embolus and suggested mitral stenosis as the cause of the pulmonary oedema.

Diagnosis and management were further complicated in this case by the history of asthma. The PEFR, carried out at the bedside, did not suggest significant reversible airway obstruction as a cause for the breathlessness. Before the cardiac diagnosis is made, many pregnant women with heart disease causing pulmonary oedema are initially labelled as having asthma. It is possible that this was also the case with Ms N. The possibility of asthma also dictated the medication used to slow her heart rate and therefore improve left-ventricular filling time (thus reducing left atrial pressure). Beta-blockers were avoided, but would have been more effective than diltiazem, a calcium-channel antagonist. Other possibilities would have been cardioselective beta-blockers, such as bisoprolol or carvedilol.

LMWH was given as recommended by Lupton et al. [43], because there was a risk of atrial fibrillation and mural thrombus.

Vaginal delivery in controlled circumstances is advocated in mitral stenosis, with careful attention to the length and normal progress of labour. A very careful epidural was given by a senior anaesthetist. Regional analgesia given slowly minimizes the risk of abrupt vasodi-lation that would be poorly tolerated in mitral stenosis. Adequate analagesia is important to limit the increased cardiac output from pain and thus reduce the risk of pulmonary oedema during the intra-partum period. LMWH administration was withheld once labour had started to ensure time for safe epidural administration. The strat-egy of fluid restriction was continued. The second stage of labour was curtailed, as recommended, by ventouse.

A further pregnancy without mitral valvotomy or valve replace-ment in this woman would be high risk, and for that reason, a plan for contraception was made, in addition to a plan for definitive treatment of the underlying cardiac disease.

5.14   SPONTANEOUS PNEUMOTHORAX

Ms P was a 29 year old nonsmoker in the 33rd week of her first preg-nancy. She attended the accident and emergency department with a 2-day history of breathlessness and chest pain. On examination, there was reduced air entry on the right and reduced chest expansion. At the time, she looked well and could talk in sentences.

A chest X-ray with abdominal shielding confirmed a large right-sided pneumothorax, with no mediastinal shift. Air (100 ml) was aspirated and she was transferred to the delivery suite. A repeat X-ray confirmed 70% expansion; a further 60 ml of air was aspirated and a chest drain was inserted. She continued to be well overnight, with oxygen saturation >97% and a respiratory rate of 31 breaths/min. She was given inspired oxygen by mask. The drain fell out, with consequent recurrence of the pneumothorax; a second drain was placed and had an underwater seal.

After 4 days, because there was a persistent air leak, pleurodesis was discussed due to the high possibility of a recurrent pneumothorax at delivery. High-volume, low-pressure suction was set up and she was transferred to the cardiothoracic ward 1 week after admission.

On day 10 after her original admission, she was taken to theatre for video-assisted thoracoscopic surgery (VATS). She was anaesthetized with a left lateral tilt. A pulmonary bleb was excised and abrasion pleurodesis was carried out. The following chest X-ray showed a small apical pneumothorax, but the drain still "bubbled" on coughing. This continued and she was transferred to the maternity unit with a Heimlich (flutter) valve rather than an underwater seal. By this time, she was at 35 weeks' gestation and all investigations on the fetus remained normal.

However, 10 days after VATS, the persistent air leak continued and a plan was made to remove the drain if the bubbling ceased for 24 hours. Furthermore, 3 weeks after the original admission, the possibility of performing talc pleurodesis was discussed because of the persistent air leak. The chest drain was, therefore, clamped and adjusted, with a reduction in the volume of the pneumothorax to <5%. Because this manoeuvre had been successful, the decision was then made to leave the chest drain in until delivery, with a plan for a further surgical procedure postpartum.

At 39 weeks' gestation, Ms P spontaneously ruptured her membranes, draining meconium-stained liquor. Following a failed stimulation of labour, she was delivered of a live male infant by emergency Caesarean section under epidural anaesthesia. The chest drain was clamped for some hours on the day after delivery, with no deterioration in symptoms. The following day, the drain was clamped for 24 hours. The drain was finally removed on day 11 postcaesarean section. A further 4 days later, she remained asymptomatic and there was no radiological evidence of pneumothorax, only pleural thickening at the apex of the right lung where the original pleurodesis was attempted.

Follow-up was planned with the chest physicians 2 weeks after discharge.

Discussion

Primary spontaneous pneumothorax is a rare complication of pregnancy, mostly occurring in the late third trimester, although sometimes at other times in pregnancy or the early postpartum period. There is a high risk of recurrence following initial resolution.

In this case, there were no obvious predisposing factors, such as smoking, either before or during pregnancy, or asthma. Ms P was of slim build, but not particularly tall. Management was in keeping with the recommendations made by the British Thoracic Society's (BTS's) latest guideline for management of primary spontaneous pneumothorax [44].

Ms P presented 2 days after onset of her symptoms, which seems to be the median time for presentation. The significance of the time lag between lung collapse and re-expansion is the risk of pulmonary oedema that can occur with re-expansion and when early suction is applied to a chest drain [44]. Here, the BTS recommendations differ from the consensus statement of the American College of Chest Physicians [45].

Because the pneumothorax was large and the patient was clinically stable, the first management measure was aspiration, followed by a repeat chest X-ray. This should be standard practice, as discussed in the BTS guideline. The pneumothorax was too large for observation alone. Again, when the lung was found not to have fully re-expanded, aspiration without recourse to a chest drain with an underwater seal was in keeping with the BTS guideline. During this time, oxygen was given by mask because this has been found to increase the reabsorption rate and improve hypoxaemia resulting from the pneumothorax [46].

Ms P needed a drain with an underwater seal once the small-bore drain had fallen out. She could equally have had a small-bore drain with a Heimlich valve inserted, giving the opportunity for outpatient management or mobilization, which was important in the prevention of thromboembolic disease, because she was in the third trimester of her pregnancy. A high-resolution CT scan could have been used at this point to image the chest and establish an underlying cause for spontaneous pneumothorax, but this would have exposed the fetus to more radiation than a plain X-ray, and several chest X-rays are likely to be requested for someone with a pneumothorax checking for resolution. The CT scan might have demonstrated underlying abnormalities and suggested the need for early surgical intervention. However, there is currently insufficient evidence to support routine use of CT, except in very specific situations [44,47].

Because of the continued air leak despite the use of an effective chest drain, the BTS guideline was followed, with two considerations in mind:

1. Definitive treatment for a protracted air leak, which was not responding to drainage with the chest drain.
2. Prevention of recurrence at the time of labour and delivery, when she was most at risk of recurrent spontaneous pneumothorax.

VATS was the treatment of choice because it enabled a good view of the lung surface, with the facility to carry out bullectomy or bleb resection, in addition to mechanical pleurodesis, an additional measure to prevent recurrence. VATS was chosen instead of talc pleurodesis because the evidence shows that VATS has a greater efficacy in preventing recurrence than talc or other forms of chemical pleurodesis because the primary cause can be located and removed [48].

Unfortunately, the VATS procedure was unsuccessful, possibly because they were unable to gain full lung re-expansion postoperatively, despite applying suction, and possibly because there was an inadequate inflammatory response to the pleurodesis procedure, perhaps due to the pregnancy. It has been suggested that VATS procedures have a higher failure rate because of a less intense pleural reaction compared with thoracotomy procedures. It is also possible that the anatomical defect responsible for the pneumothorax was not identified and removed. At this point, the small-bore chest drain with the Heimlich valve was used. Unfortunately, despite the possibility of being treated as an out-patient, Ms P no longer had the confidence to go home with the chest drain in situ, having been in hospital for 2 weeks by this time.

The decision was finally made to allow her to labour with the chest drain in situ because this was the safest option and the concern about curtailing the second stage of labour due to the risk of recurrence would be avoided. This was followed by spontaneous resolution in the immediate postpartum period.

By its very nature, management of this condition requires that several chest X-rays be carried out to demonstrate resolution. In this woman, some of these X-rays were performed in the delivery suite using portable equipment that produced antero posterior (AP) films. Because of the potential risks to the fetus of ionizing radiation (i.e. an increased risk of malignancy in later life) [47], it might have been wiser to try as far as possible to have all films taken in the X-ray department because this ensures that the lowest dose of radiation possible is given to the mother and fetus. By definition, the portable film increases exposure because of the position of the patient, the equipment itself, the difficulty in the patient holding her breath in expiration and the need for extended exposure time [47]. This should encourage departmental X-rays, where possible. However, the risk from chest X-rays is very low, whether portable or within the department, because the radiation dose is small, being equivalent to only a few days of background irradiation. Chest X-rays that are clinically indicated should never be withheld because of pregnancy.

Although CT has been suggested to have a limited role in the management of pneumothorax, the type of CT has not been elucidated. Spiral CT, as used in the diagnosis of pulmonary embolus, will afford reduced radiation doses, but it could be that high-resolution CT is more appropriate for the investigation of pneumothorax, particularly secondary pneumothorax.

It is difficult to know whether chemical pleurodesis would have given success in this case, when mechanical pleurodesis did not. The only other procedure that could have been considered to prevent a recurrence of pneumothorax is pleurectomy, either at the time of the VATS procedure or through open thoracotomy. Chemical pleurodesis is known to have reduced efficacy, compared with VATS, for prevention of recurrence and is also associated with particular dangers. Doxycycline, a tetracycline, could not have been used in this patient because she was pregnant and there is a potential risk of discolouration of fetal teeth and bones. With talc pleurodesis, there is a potential risk of empyema and acute adult respiratory distress syndrome (ARDS), especially with doses above 5 g [44].

Finally, the question of whether an adequate sterile inflammation would develop in a pregnant patient remains unaddressed in the literature.

5.15 SEVERE PRE-ECLAMPSIA AND HAEMOLYTIC URAEMIC SYNDROME

Mrs Q was a 26 year old, black African nurse booked-in during her first ongoing pregnancy. She had a normal booking blood pressure of 100/60 mmHg and normal booking investigations, including a full infection screen that was negative. She remained well until 25 weeks' gestation, when she was admitted from the antenatal clinic with a blood pressure of 190/108 mmHg, 4+ proteinuria and 2+ blood in her urine. She also said she had passed less urine during the preceding 3 days and was complaining of headache, nausea and vomiting.

Mrs Q was admitted and therapy with methyldopa, 500 mg three times daily was commenced. A 24-hour urinary protein collection of 528 ml was analysed and found to have a protein excretion rate of 15.75 g/24 hours. Her MSU, which was sent that day, was negative. Other results of note were as follows: platelet count, 275×10^9

platelets/l; creatinine, 63 μmol/l; albumin, 27 g/l; and urate, 0.32 mmol/l. With the diagnosis of pre-eclampsia confirmed, the plan was for continued in-patient management and delivery for the usual fetal or maternal indications.

After 5 days, Mrs Q awoke with a severe frontal headache and blood pressure of 198/110 mmHg; she was also complaining of severe blurring of vision and epigastric pain. There was no vaginal bleeding. The CTG trace at this point was also suspicious, with recurrent, unprovoked, shallow decelerations. She was transferred to the obstetric high-dependency unit, for stabilization before delivery, and the pre-eclampsia protocol was commenced. She was given a preload of 500 ml of colloid and then bolus doses of hydralazine and MgSO$_4$ (4 g), followed by a MgSO$_4$ infusion of 1 g/hour. Within 30 minutes, she was found to be coughing up pink frothy sputum. On examination, she had a raised JVP and bilateral basal inspiratory crepitations, suggesting pulmonary oedema. She was treated with a 40 mg intravenous bolus of frusemide. Blood results, from serum taken that morning, were then obtained. These showed creatinine of 126 μm/l, albumin of 18 g/l (the previous day's result was 24 g/l), bilirubin of 30 μm/l and urate of 0.4 mmol/l. Her platelet count had dropped to 108×10^9 platelets/l. The serum potassium value was unavailable because the sample was thought to be haemolysed. The MgSO$_4$ infusion was stopped because of anuria. Fetal demise was also confirmed at this time by ultrasound scan, once the heart trace was lost on the CTG.

An urgent ultrasound of the renal tract excluded renal vein thrombosis and showed normal-size kidneys, but suggested diffuse parenchymal renal disease. She was given misoprostol per vagina, followed by oral misoprostol 3 hours later. By this time, her serum urea level was 7.5 mmol/l and her creatinine level was 189 μmol/l.

By the following morning, her creatinine level had risen to 273 μmol/l and her urea level had risen to 10.3 mmol/l. The Hb concentration was 8.5 g/dl and the platelet count was 40×10^9 platelets/l. A blood film showed burr cells, fragmented red cells, spherocytes and normal platelets, suggesting a microangiopathic coagulopathy. At that point, a reticulocyte count, direct Coombs' antibody test (DAT) and serum antibodies were requested.

Despite the rising creatinine level and oliguria, her serum potassium level was not raised. Her liver function remained normal, but her serum albumin level dropped to 16 g/l. The expectation was that once the fetus was delivered, which occurred 3 hours later, renal function would improve. This was also the opinion of the renal physician that morning.

Unfortunately, despite vaginal delivery of a 960 g male fetus, her renal function continued to deteriorate over the next 36 hours: her creatinine level was 791 μm/l, her urea level was 23.5 mmol/l and her serum potassium level was 6.0 mmol/l. The anaemia and thrombocytopenia had also worsened: her Hb concentration was 6.7 g/dl, her haematocrit was 0.197 and her platelet count was 34×10^9 platelets/l. Treatment for hyperkalaemia was instituted with actrapid insulin, glucose and calcium resonium (15 g orally). Once the serum potassium level had fallen to 5.1 mmol/l, 2 days after delivery, Mrs Q was transferred to the renal unit.

On the renal unit, she was treated with plasmapheresis on five occasions and had two episodes of dialysis. With the last four treatments of plasmapheresis, she was given chlorpheniramine and hydrocortisone because she had a severe allergic reaction to the first treatment.

She was discharged 10 days later with a creatinine level of 191 μmmol/l and on the following medication:

Doxazocin, 8 mg twice daily
Nifedipine modified release, 20 mg twice daily
Bisoprolol, 10 mg once daily
Sandocal, 1 tablet twice daily

Her blood pressure was well controlled on these drugs and she remained under the care of the renal physicians for follow-up.

Discussion

Haemolytic uraemic syndrome (HUS) is a constellation of three clinical features, as follows:

Microangiopathic haemolytic anaemia (DAT negative)
Thrombocytopenia
Renal failure [49]

HUS can be further divided into diarrhoeal and nondiarrhoeal subtypes; the diarrhoeal form is seen most commonly in children and adults in association with bacterial gastrointestinal infection, notably with *Escherichia coli* 0157. HUS is thought to develop because of the verocytotoxin produced by the interaction of *E. coli* with a lipopolysaccharide co-factor [49]. It is a very rare condition, related to thrombotic thrombocytopenic purpura (TTP), with an incidence of 3.7 cases per million (in adults) [50]. In pregnancy, it is thought to occur 3–10 weeks postpartum [51].

Nondiarrhoeal HUS can be familial or sporadic. In the familial form, there are autosomal dominant and autosomal recessive patterns of inheritance [49].

Sporadic HUS can be associated with a number of factors, such as the following:

Pregnancy
SLE
Antiphospholipid syndrome
HIV
The combined oral contraceptive pill (COCP)
Ciclosporin

In Mrs Q, pregnancy was obviously an issue, but SLE or other autoantibody condition could have been contributory [52]. Interestingly, Mrs Q subsequently tested positive for both anticardiolipin antibodies and lupus anticoagulant and had a high (1/1280) antinuclear antibody (ANA) titre.

HUS in this case declared itself at the time of delivery but it has also been described in the first trimester. If, as in this case, HUS occurs immediately postpartum or in the third trimester of pregnancy, the following differential diagnoses, or associated conditions, must be excluded:

HELLP syndrome
AFLP
TTP

In both AFLP and HELLP syndrome, liver function tests are abnormal; however, abnormal liver function tests are unusual in HUS and TTP. TTP can be more difficult to differentiate clinically, although it causes a more widespread thrombotic angiopathy, often with neurological symptoms.

Nondiarrhoeal HUS is thought to be due to a deficiency or mutation in the gene coding for factor H, a complement regulator. As a result, low complement C3 levels might be a feature, although they are not always. Because of the absence or deficiency of this factor, it could be that the alternative complement pathway cannot be activated to interrupt the clotting cascade once endothelial damage has occurred.

The following treatments have been described as effective in the literature:

Plasmapheresis
Antithrombin infusions
Prostacyclin infusions
Immunoglobulin (Ig) after failed plasmapheresis and plasma replacement [51].

The mainstay of therapy is now plasmapheresis, and platelet transfusion is contraindicated, because it can exacerbate rather than ameliorate the condition. Currently, it is unclear why plasmapheresis works in HUS. It might help to remove large platelet aggregates and might, in some way, help to control or reduce further platelet agglutination.

Although the differential diagnosis, especially between HELLP syndrome and HUS, is often difficult, this case was relatively clear-cut because there was little liver dysfunction, thereby excluding AFLP and HELLP syndrome. There were no focal neurological symptoms, making TTP unlikely, and renal dysfunction seemed to be out of proportion to the pre-eclampsia. Until relatively recently, HUS had a high mortality rate (of >60%). Thankfully, the advent of plasmapheresis has reduced this considerably. However, for Mrs Q, careful counselling is required concerning the next pregnancy.

5.16 HYPERSPLENISM

Mrs R was a 28 year old black, African woman, who booked in her first pregnancy at 9 weeks' gestation. She was fit and well, apart from splenomegaly, for which she had undergone extensive investigation during the previous year. She was known to have sickle cell trait and received appropriate counselling from the haemaglobinopathy specialist nurse counsellor. Her partner was sickle cell negative. Her other booking results confirmed that she was negative for HIV 1 and 2, and that she was a low infectivity carrier of hepatitis B. After a consultation with the consultant virologist, her partner was vaccinated and arrangements were set in place for the baby to be treated after birth. Results of the booking full blood count showed a platelet count of 38×10^9 platelets/l, a Hb concentration of 11.9 g/dl and that there was relative leucopenia.

Splenomegaly was first detected by her GP, before this pregnancy, when she attended the surgery complaining of constipation. During the examination, the spleen was palpable five fingerbreadths below the left costal margin. She was referred to a gastroenterologist and investigated over a 12-month period (Table 5.4).

It was felt that splenomegaly was secondary to a previous malarial infection and no further action was taken, apart from regular follow-up.

After the finding of thrombocytopenia in pregnancy, a trial of prednisolone (20 mg for 2 weeks) was given in the hope that the platelet count might rise. However, the platelet count remained between 31×10^9 platelets/l and 53×10^9 platelets/l, and thus prednisolone was stopped. The clinical haematologists became involved in her care and suggested that splenectomy should be considered following delivery, to allow the platelet level to rise. The pregnancy continued uneventfully, with Hb levels within the normal range for pregnancy and no evidence of haemolysis. There were no episodes of bruising, vaginal bleeding or epistaxis during the pregnancy.

TABLE 5.4. Results of investigations for splenomegaly

Upper abdominal ultrasound	Normal liver, no ascites. Spleen 19 cm with normal uniform texture
Brucella serology	Negative
Malaria	Negative
Abdominal CT scan	Confirmed normal liver, with normal portal circulation, and normal kidneys. Massively enlarged spleen with no focal abnormality
G6PD assay	Negative
Reticulocyte count	Normal, with normal ferritin levels
FBC	Hb, 13.2 g/dl; WBC, 7.6 × 10^9/l; platelet count, 44 × 10^9 platelets/l
Clotting	INR, 1.18; APTT, 1.07 (both with 50/50 correction) Fibrinogen, 1.48 g/l
Bone marrow	Normal

APTT - activated partial thromboplastin time; CT - computed tomography; FBC - full blood count; G6PD - glucose 6 phosphate dehydrogenase; Hb - haemoglobin; INR - international normalized ratio; WBC - white blood cells.

The plan for labour included taking samples for a full blood count and crossmatching two units of blood on admission, and establishing intravenous access. A consultant obstetric anaesthetist counselled that regional anaesthesia was contraindicated if the platelet count was below 80 × 10^9 platelets/l and suggested that Entonox and intravenous opioids could be used for analgesia in labour. General anaesthesia was recommended in the event of an emergency Caesarean section. It was also noted that NSAIDs should not be used for analgesia and that intramuscular injections should be avoided.

At 41 weeks' gestation, a membrane sweep was carried out. She was admitted at 41 + 3 weeks' gestation for induction of labour. The Hb concentration was 11.9 g/dl and the platelet count was 54 × 10^9 platelets/l when induction was commenced. She laboured after receiving 5 mg of intravaginal prostin in divided doses. Unfortunately, an emergency Caesarean section was necessary at 8 cm dilatation, for suspected fetal distress. Free fluid was noted at the time of the Caesarean. A live female infant was delivered, weighing 3.13 kg. The estimated blood loss was 750 ml and an infusion of Syntocinon (40 iu) was commenced at a rate of 10 iu/hour. A negative pressure drain was placed at the time of surgery, which drained 370 ml in the first 24 hours and, subsequently, a further 870 ml of serosanguinous fluid. Postpartum ultrasound confirmed the presence of ascites and revealed that the splenic size had reduced from a maximum of 21 cm to 12 cm. On the first day postcaesarean section, she was found to be anaemic with a Hb concentration of 8.8 g/dl and a platelet count of 38×10^9 platelets/l; iron was prescribed. The drain was removed and she was discharged on the fifth postoperative day, with arrangements for haematology and gastroenterology follow-up appointments.

Discussion

"Hypersplenism" is a term used to describe splenomegaly, from any cause, and its consequences.

The causes of splenomegaly include the following:
Infection
Inflammation
Haematological
Miscellaneous

A greatly enlarged spleen is more common in the presence of myelofibrosis, chronic leukaemia, chronic malaria, kala-azar or Gaucher's disease (lysosomal storage disease). Chronic malaria was felt to be the cause of splenomegaly in this case, although no evidence of malarial parasites had ever been found. Other infectious causes had been excluded, including hepatitis. Although Mrs R was known to be hepatitis B positive, she was shown to be of low infectivity and did not have evidence of chronic hepatitis [53]. There was no evidence of investigation for sarcoidosis, another recognised cause for hypersplenism [54].

Hypersplenism can result in pancytopenia, haemolysis and an increased plasma volume, but the only features present during pregnancy in Mrs R were thrombocytopenia and intermittent leucopenia, which had been evident before pregnancy.

When she was first seen by the obstetrician, her previous medical notes were unavailable. The first thought was that the thrombocytopenia was caused by immune thrombocytopenic pupura (ITP), because the count was lower than expected for gestational thrombocytopenia at 20 weeks' gestation. It was known that Mrs R was HIV 1 and 2 negative and that she did not have lupus anticoagulant or anticardiolipin anibodies. Antiplatelet antibodies were not assayed, because they were considered unlikely to change management. There was no evidence of SLE. The platelet count was checked using a citrate sample, which confirmed that it was a true thrombocytopenia, rather than a spurious result due to in-vitro platelet clumping.

A trial of prednisolone was given to promote a rise in the platelet count, assuming the low count was related to an immunological cause. The platelet count did not rise and prednisolone was stopped. It could be argued that immune thrombocytopenia was not adequately excluded because the steroid trial was not at a dose high enough to bring about a response. The usual treatment for suspected refractory ITP is prednisolone at a dose of 1 mg/kg body weight, but this is often associated with relapse. A dose equivalent to 250 mg of prednisolone over 4 days has been recommended [55] and found to produce a sustained rise in the platelet count; however, this runs the significant risk of side effects, such as mood swings, steroid psychosis, hypertension and deranged glucose metabolism, all of which would be best avoided in pregnancy.

It was appropriate to make appointments for a predelivery anaesthetic opinion, both to give the obstetric anaesthetic staff warning of this high-risk patient and to allow the patient to be fully informed of her choices and the potential difficulties surrounding delivery and analgesia. It meant that when an emergency caesarean was carried out, she was emotionally and mentally prepared, and the unit was prepared with crossmatched blood and intravenous access. The haematologists should have been informed when she went into labour, because of the possibility of needing platelet cover during delivery, if her platelets had dropped low enough ($<20 \times 10^9$ platelets/l) [56]. In fact, at the time of induction (which was carried out because she was approaching 42 weeks of completed gestation), her platelet level was $>50 \times 10^9$ platelets/l, a level at which she was not expected to be at higher risk of bleeding, although it still precluded regional anaesthesia.

Fetal blood sampling was avoided because Mrs R was known to be hepatitis B positive and fetal thrombocytopenia remained a possibility. Her blood pressure during labour was around 140/80 mmHg, compared with a booking blood pressure of 94/60 mmHg, and it is noteworthy that there was a degree of renal impairment, with the creatinine level rising from 71 μmol/l in the mid-trimester to 138 μmol/l peripartum. This was associated with a rise in bilirubin 26 μmol/l and ALT 180 iu/l, which together with an additional fall in the platelet count and a drop in the Hb concentration greater than expected for the estimated blood loss, suggested HELLP syndrome; there was no record of proteinuria or urinalysis during labour, but this does not preclude the diagnosis. Alternatively, the rise in creatinine might have been related to postpartum haemorrhage and the rise in ALT might have been related to the usual physiological postpartum effect, although both changes were more marked than is usually seen in those circumstances.

The cause of the splenomegaly remains unresolved in this case, although the new finding of ascites might help future investigations. The platelet count is one of the factors that will determine management, including the need for splenectomy.

5.17 SPINA BIFIDA WITH SEVERE KYPHOSCOLIOSIS

Mrs S was a 31 year old para 1 + 0 who attended the medical obstetric clinic at 10 weeks' gestation with an unplanned pregnancy.

She had spina bifida diagnosed at birth and underwent repair of two large thoraco-lumbar lesions, with subsequent surgery on several occasions as an infant. She had very severe kyphoscoliosis, but did not report any bladder or bowel problems nor suffer from recurrent urinary tract infections.

Mrs S had had one previous pregnancy and reported that an elective Caesarean section had been performed at 34 weeks' gestation because "the baby ran out of room". That pregnancy had been planned and she had attended for prepregnancy counselling and had pulmonary function tests performed before conception. These indicated that the forced vital capacity (FVC) was 1.21 l, resting blood gases were normal and overnight oximetry showed no desaturation. There was no evidence of incipient respiratory failure, but the respiratory reserve was very limited. She was strongly encouraged to stop smoking, which she succeeded in doing. An echocardiogram showed no evidence of secondary pulmonary hypertension.

During that previous pregnancy, she had presented for booking at 14 weeks' gestation and was taking folic acid (5 mg) at conception. She had early dating and nuchal translucency scans, which were normal, in addition to a fetal anomaly scan at 20 weeks' gestation, which was also normal. The respiratory physicians, obstetrician and the medical obstetric team saw her regularly. The respiratory team arranged a trial of nasal intermittent positive airways ventilation (NIPPV) on an in-patient basis at 30 weeks' gestation and she tolerated this very well. Overnight oximetry was performed at home at 31 weeks' gestation, with no evidence of desaturation.

She had become increasingly breathless at 32 weeks' gestation and could only walk 20 m without stopping because of severe breathlessness. She was admitted to the antenatal ward for rest. Further sleep testing showed deterioration in her oxygen saturation and it was decided to deliver her by elective Caesarean section at 34 weeks' gestation. A female infant was delivered without complications. Mrs S was initially admitted to the intensive care unit (ICU) postoperatively and NIPPV was required for several days postdelivery. The baby remained in SCBU for a few days, and at the time of presentation in the second pregnancy, she was a fit and healthy 4 year old. Mrs S returned to her prepregnancy function level within a few days.

On this occasion, Mrs S had been using condoms for contraception, and because this was an unplanned pregnancy, she had commenced

5 mg of folic acid only on confirmation of a positive pregnancy test, at approximately 8 weeks' gestation. She was keen to proceed with the pregnancy and thus an early dating scan and first trimester screening tests were organized. Pulmonary function tests and an echocardiogram were arranged. Mrs S was warned that there might have been some deterioration in her pulmonary capacity since her previous pregnancy and that the likelihood was of a similar pregnancy course, with admission necessary during the third trimester and early delivery by Caesarean section. She was concerned by this possibility and the necessary frequent visits to hospital, because this would have an impact on her daughter.

Discussion

Mrs S was born with diastematomyelia, also termed "split cord malformation", which is a form of occult spinal dysraphism characterized by a cleft in the spinal column. It can be isolated or associated with other dysraphisms, segmental anomalies of the vertebral bodies or visceral malformations – horseshoe or ectopic kidney, utero-ovarian malformation and anorectal malformation. It is rare, but the neonatal outcome of isolated diastematomyelia is generally good, even if surgical repair is required.

The issues relating to pregnancy in these patients include the following:

Genetic counselling – any female patient with spina bifida is strongly recommended to have preconceptual genetic counselling. For parents with spina bifida, the risk of having affected offspring is approximately 4%, which is considerably increased compared with the general population (in which the risk is 0.1–0.3% [57]). This risk can be lowered if periconceptual folic acid is given.

Potential urological complications include neurogenic bladder, incontinence, chronic infection, an increased risk of developing bladder carcinoma and impaired renal function, and are common in spina bifida. In cases of urinary diversion, obstruction could complicate the pregnancy. The risk of recurrent urinary tract infection is increased, especially if there is a history of recurrent urinary tract infection outside pregnancy – a careful and detailed history must be taken at the initial booking appointment.

The incidence of preterm labour is increased, in addition to cephalo-pelvic disproportion because of a possibly contracted pelvis – this can be assessed to a limited extent using CT or MRI scanning. Transverse lie is common, but if the head engages normally, vaginal delivery should be allowed, if possible.

Cerebrospinal fluid shunts could produce neurological problems during pregnancy. In most reported cases, symptoms improved spontaneously after delivery. In a woman with a shunt, vaginal delivery is preferable, pushing during the second stage of labour is not contraindicated and, for a Caesarean section, prophylactic antibiotics and thorough irrigation of the peritoneal cavity are indicated.

A large case series describes 29 pregnancies in 17 women, with 23 pregnancies progressing to births [58]. Of the 17 women, 14 women had antenatal admissions, with wheelchair-dependent women requiring more frequent and longer admissions. Recurrent urinary tract infection occurred in women with a prior history of urinary infection. Mobility was reduced for two women during pregnancy, with a full recovery afterwards. Pre-existing pressure sores worsened during pregnancy. Vaginal deliveries occurred in 20% of wheelchair-dependent women and in 55% of independently mobile women. Caesarean sections had a high postoperative complication rate.

The problem of kyphoscoliosis in pregnancy is uncommon: the literature since 1996 describes only 36 cases [59].

Women with severe lung disease are less likely to deteriorate in pregnancy than those with severe cardiac disease. Figures, such as 1 1 or 50% of predicted FVC, have been suggested for successful pregnancy outcome. However, women with much lower FVC have had successful pregnancies. Further deterioration in lung function as a result of the pregnancy can be expected, and in women with a FVC of 1–1.5 l, severe limitations in exercise capacity, fatigue and hypersomnolence are expected. Pulmonary hypertension should be excluded with a prepregnancy echocardiogram. There are case reports in the literature of NIPPV with bilevel positive airway pressure used to correct exercise tolerance, fatigue and nocturnal oxygen desaturation [60]. This was trialled in Mrs S, although it was not required until the immediate postpartum period.

Anaesthetic review is essential as part of delivery planning.

5.18 PEMPHIGOID GESTATIONIS

Ms T was a 24 year old primigravid patient from the Middle East who booked at 13 weeks' gestation. Her booking bloods were normal, with no evidence of a haemoglobinopathy. Her Hb concentration was

11.2 g/dl and her booking blood pressure was recorded as 110/75 mmHg.

There was no contributory past medical history. She had been well throughout the pregnancy, until presenting at 29 weeks' gestation with a rash. On examination, she had pruritic erythematous, urticarial plaques and vesicles on her hands, extremities, trunk, face and scalp. There was no history of any drug ingestion, hormonal therapy or any systemic symptoms.

A skin biopsy was performed under local anaesthetic, which showed positive complement C3 linear basement-membrane staining with direct immunofluorescence and positive staining to IgG and complement C3 under indirect immunofluorescence. Therefore, a diagnosis of pemphigoid gestationis was made. Therapy was commenced with prednisolone, 60 mg/day, topical betamethasone cream and antihistamines. Over the next month, her condition improved. A preterm, healthy baby boy was delivered vaginally at 34 weeks' gestation. However, during his first week of life, he developed multiple erythematous urticarial plaques and bullae, which responded well to a low-potency steroid cream.

In the puerperium, Ms T developed a flare, for which she was treated with prednisolone, 80 mg/day, chlorpheniramine, 4 mg three times daily, and fucidin and betnovate creams. Additional treatment included ciclosporin, 300 mg/day, intravenous Ig (two courses), pulsed intravenous methylprednisolone, mycophenolate mofetil, 3 g/day, and azathioprine, 200 mg daily.

At 10 months postpartum, she again developed widespread blisters on erythrematous itchy plaques, which showed positive IgG linear basement-membrane staining. Investigations performed at this stage showed the following:

C-reactive protein:	55 g/l
Albumin:	29 g/l
Hb:	10.3 g/dl
Eosinophils:	1.6×10^9/l
Autoantibody screen:	negative

A hormone profile and glucose test were both normal. A chest X-ray was normal and a dual X ray absorpitometry (DEXA) bone-density scan revealed osteopenia. The following treatment was commenced: methylprednisolone, 1 g/day intravenously for 3 days; Ig, 2 g/kg body weight intravenously over 3 days; prednisolone, 50 mg/day; mycophenolate mofetil, 3.5 g/day; Atarax, 25 mg/day; ranitidine, 150 mg/day; alendronate, 70 mg once weekly; Calcichew, 2 tablets/day; antiseptic soaks; and emollients. Over the ensuing months she made a full recovery.

Discussion

Pemphigoid gestationis is a rare condition that can complicate 1 out of 40,000–60,000 pregnancies. It was initially named "herpes gestationis" by Milton in 1872, which comes from the Greek "to creep". This is, however, a misnomer because the disease is not related to any active or prior herpes infection. Jenkins et al. have argued for the term "pemphigoid gestationis" [61].

Pemphigoid gestationis is a pregnancy-associated autoimmune disease. Most patients develop antibodies to the basement-membrane protein bullous pemphigoid antigen 2 (BPAG2; collagen XVII), which has a crucial role in epidermal–dermal adhesion. Binding of IgG to the basement membrane is believed to trigger an immune response that leads to the formation of subepidermal vesicles and blisters. The same antibodies occur in patients with bullous pemphigoid (BP) [62].

The trigger for development of autoantibodies remains elusive. Crossreactivity between placental tissue and skin has been proposed to have a role. Pemphigoid gestationis has a strong association with HLA-DR3 and HLA-DR4, and virtually all patients with a history of pemphigoid gestationis have demonstrable anti-HLA antibodies. The placenta is known to be the main source of disparate (paternal) antibodies and thus can present an immunological target during gestation.

Pemphigoid gestationis typically occurs in the second to third trimester, with 50–75% of affected women experiencing a postpartum flare within 24–48 hours of delivery [63]. Classically, it presents as pruritic erythematous, urticated papules and plaques (which might appear target-like, annular or polycyclic) and could develop into vesicles/tense blisters within days or a few weeks. The rash usually starts in the periumbilical area (90%).

Pemphigoid gestationis is a dermatosis specific to pregnancy, in addition to polymorphic eruption of pregnancy (PEP), prurigo of pregnancy and pruritic folliculitis, from which it can usually be easily differentiated [64]. The differential diagnoses include other autoimmune bullous diseases, drug eruptions and erythema multiforme.

Diagnosis is made by direct immunofluorescence, which shows positive complement C3 deposition at the basement membrane. IgG titres do not correlate to disease activity.

Prognosis for the initial presentation is good, but recurrences are common (as demonstrated by this case), especially postpartum, and can occur with oral contraceptive use, the menstrual cycle and, less commonly, ovulation. The disease could persist for anything from a couple of weeks to several years postpartum. There is a reported case of active disease 12 years postpartum [63].

There is a high risk of recurrence in subsequent pregnancies, unless the partner is changed. Recurrences tend to occur at an earlier gestational age and with increased severity. Because there are immunological factors implicated in the pathogenesis, fetal and/or neonatal disease is a logical possibility. There is debate in the literature about overall fetal outcome, but generally it is accepted that 5–10% of babies present with transient urticarial or vesicular lesions, which resolve spontaneously in 2–3 weeks (as in this case). Some studies have shown an increased incidence of prematurity and small-for-date babies; therefore, regular ultrasound surveillance is suggested [63]. There is no apparent increase in the long-term risk of other autoimmune diseases.

Pemphigoid gestationis is associated with HLA-DR3 and HLA-DR4, in addition to trophoblastic tumours (choriocarcinoma and hydatidiform mole), Graves' disease, Hashimoto's thyroiditis, pernicious anaemia, Crohn's disease, alopecia areata, and antithyroid and antiplatelet antibodies.

This case is unusual, because there was a recurrence of symptoms 10 months after the postpartum recurrence. Because there is an overlap between these bullous diseases, it is conceivable that this actually represented a conversion from pemphigus gestationis to bullous pemphigoid, which has been previously reported [61].

5.19 TAKAYASU'S ARTERITIS

Mrs V was a 29 year old nulliparous Asian woman who presented to the obstetric medicine clinic for prepregnancy counselling. She had been diagnosed with Takayasu's arteritis 8 years previously but was told her disease was now quiescent. She was asymptomatic and taking prednisolone, 5 mg/day. Both radial and brachial pulses were absent on the left, but using auscultation over the right brachial artery, her blood pressure was 132/76 mmHg.

Discussion

Takayasu's arteritis is a disease of heterogeneous manifestation, progression and response to treatment. It is characterized by acute attacks of pulseless large-vessel arteritis, followed by stenosis, most commonly of the aorta and its branches above and below the diaphragm. Following clinical assessment, the diagnosis is made using angiography, duplex ultrasound scanning and/or MRI. There are no reliable biochemical markers of disease activity, and C-reactive protein and ESR are not helpful in initial diagnosis or assessment of relapse. Fulfilment of three of the six diagnostic criteria is necessary for the diagnosis of Takayasu's arteritis, as proposed by the American College of Rheumatology (ACR) in 1990 (Table 5.5). Table 5.6 describes the anatomical angiographic classification adapted from the Takayasu Conference of 1994.

Asian people are more commonly affected than other ethnic groups, regardless of their country of residence. It is a rare condition, with a prevalence of 2 in 1 million individuals in the UK. The mean age of diagnosis is 25 years, and 70% of patients are female. Hence, the commonest patient group is women of reproductive age. However, it also occurs in children. A monophasic attack with residual stenotic *sequelae* is exhibited by 20% of patients. Half of these patients go into remission with immunosuppressive therapy, but 50% of these treated patients relapse within 5 years. A further 30% of these patients have progressive disease that is unresponsive to therapy. Although the 10-year survival rate is >90%, 75% of patients suffer significant morbidity, affecting their daily life. Cardiac failure is the most common cause of death.

Clinical symptoms depend on the site, and extent, of pathology and are attributed to end-organ ischaemia. Feeble or absent peripheral

TABLE 5.5.   Modified American College of Rheumatology diagnostic criteria, 1990 for Takayasu's arteritis

1. Development of symptoms or signs before 40 years of age.
2. Claudication of extremeties, fatigue or discomfort on use of limbs.
3. Decreased brachial artery pulse, either unilateral or bilateral.
4. Blood pressure difference of at least 10 mmHg between arms.
5. Audible bruit over subclavian artery or abdominal aorta.
6. Angiogram abnormalities: stenosis or occlusion of aorta, its main branches or large vessels in proximal upper and lower extremities, which is not caused by atherosclerosis.

Table 5.6. Angiographic classification for Takayasu's arteritis

Type	Site of disease
Type I	Only branches of aortic arch
Type IIa	Ascending aorta and above
Type IIb	Descending thoracic aorta and above
Type III	Thoracic, abdominal and/or renal
Type IV	Abdominal and/or renal
Type V	Mix of types IIb and IV

pulses, with resultant claudication, with or without bruits are hall-marks of the disease. Bruits are the most common clinical sign, present in 80% of patients. These are most commonly heard over the carotid arteries, which are involved in 60% of patients, of which 60% have bilateral disease. Carotidynia is present in up to 30% of patients. Cardiovascular pathology is present in 40% of patients, most commonly aortic regurgitation. Pulmonary hypertension is present in 5% of patients. Systemic and renovascular hypertension develops in 75% of patients. Other complications include cardiac insufficiency and stroke. Systemic symptoms of lethargy and fatigue are present in 40% of patients, and about 25% of patients have significant pyrexia during acute episodes. Ophthalmological and neurological symptoms warrant aggressive assessment and urgent treatment [65,66,67].

Ishikawa suggested a clinical classification, grouping 54 patients into 4 categories according to the site and severity of disease (Table 5.7). Ishikawa gave importance to four main complications, namely retinopathy, secondary hypertension, aortic regurgitation and aneurysm formation. Most of the fatalities occurred in groups II and III. All patients with aortic regurgitation were classified as group IIB. However, this system of classification is not applicable to pregnant women, because pulmonary hypertension carries a 30–50% mortality in pregnancy.

There have been various series reporting an association between Takayasu's arteritis and tuberculosis. These series are mainly from Asia, where the prevalence of tuberculosis is high and it is difficult to prove causality.

NSAIDs are used during acute attacks to alleviate symptoms, but the main treatment option is corticosteroids. In 50% of cases, steroids alone fail to achieve remission and adjuvant immunosuppressive agents are added to the regimen; the most commonly used immunosupressive agents are methotrexate, cyclophosphamide and azathioprine. No one agent is superior to another in achieving disease remission. Surgical grafting of critically stenosed vessels is indicated in the following situations:

Severe renovascular hypertension.

Table 5.7. Ishikawa classification 1978 for Takayasu's arteritis

Group I	Uncomplicated disease, with or without pulmonary involvement
Group IIA	Mild/moderate single complication with uncomplicated disease
Group IIB	Single severe complication
Group III	Two or more complications

Significant (symptomatic) cerebral ischaemia, with a minimum of three-vessel involvement.

Grade II aortic regurgitation.

Coronary insufficiency.

Claudication of extremities.

Almost one-third of surgical procedures have significant complications, including restenosis in 25% of these [68].

It is not uncommon for Takayasu's arteritis to present for the first time in pregnancy. Indeed, this was the main route of patient recruitment in some series. Because pregnancy is rare among women with severe disease, favourable pregnancy outcomes have been reported in many series. One study observed that pregnancy seems to confer a prognostic advantage, but this is likely to be due to the fact that women with milder forms of the disease conceive.

Pregnancy itself does not seem to affect the course or prognosis of the disease, and the risk of relapse does not seem to be increased, even in the postpartum period. Pregnancy, however, might mask and delay the diagnosis of Takayasu's arteritis. Fatigue, lethargy, headaches, light-headedness, calf cramps and cardiac murmurs are all inherent to pregnancy. Furthermore, there might be temptation to delay diagnostic testing in pregnancy for fear of fetal radiation exposure. Duplex ultrasound scanning and MRI are safe alternatives to angiography, with negligible fetal risks. Steroid therapy must be continued in pregnancy if clinically indicated.

Monitoring of disease could pose a clinical challenge. Angiography is relatively contraindicated. The ESR is raised in pregnancy, and both the ESR and the C-reactive protein level are nonspecific disease markers. The hyperdynamic circulation of pregnancy can make bruits louder, giving a false sense of disease progression. Blood pressure measurement should ideally be performed on an unaffected limb. However, this might be difficult and even impossible if all four limbs are involved.

There might be deterioration of cardiac and renal function during pregnancy. The risks are proportional to the degree of prepregnancy insufficiency.

The worst outcomes are usually in women with cardiac insufficiency, severe hypertension and significant aortic regurgitation, for which the risks of miscarriage, IUGR, prematurity, intrauterine death (IUD) and Caesarean section are increased. The risk of preeclampsia is increased with renovascular hypertension. Fetal or neonatal arteritis has not been described.

Outcomes are favourable if pregnancy is conceived during a quiescent phase or if the maintenance immunosuppressive regimen is ≤ 5 mg of prednisolone on alternate days.

Complications that must be addressed before embarking on pregnancy include cardiac insufficiency, severe renovascular hypertension, aortic regurgitation and renal insufficiency. Pregnancy is contraindicated in the presence of pulmonary hypertension and significant cardiac insufficiency.

Steroid therapy is safe in pregnancy. However, the commonly used immunosuppressive agents methotrexate and cyclophosphamide are contraindicated because they cause pregnancy loss and are teratogenic. Azathioprine seems to be safe in pregnancy and breastfeeding. Acute inflammation can pose a therapeutic challenge because long-term use of NSAIDs beyond 24 weeks' gestation has been associated with oligohydramnios and premature closure of the ductus arteriosus. Short-term use before 32 weeks' gestation is permissible with monitoring of liquor volume and, if feasible, Doppler assessment of ductus arteriosus flow. Oligohydramnios is an indication to stop treatment, following which there is usually spontaneous restoration of liquor volume.

The patient with Takayasu's arteritis who wishes to embark on pregnancy should ideally be seen in the prepregnancy clinic setting. A planned pregnancy is vital because the outcome is determined by the lack of active disease at conception. Disease-suppressive or disease-modifying drugs must be reviewed, and if necessary, changed to an alternative therapy that is less damaging to the fetus. Hypertension must be controlled with agents that are not teratogenic. Severe stenoses should be surgically corrected before pregnancy. Aneurysms, especially cerebral, should be sought and treatment considered before pregnancy. Severe uncorrected aortic regurgitation is also a relative contraindication to pregnancy. Steroid-induced diabetes should be controlled. Women with hypertension should be counselled concerning the increased risk of pre-eclampsia. Women with mild quiescent disease should not be discouraged from pregnancy because outcomes are favourable.

Pregnancy should be managed by a multidisciplinary team who are familiar with high-risk pregnancies, including a physician, obstetrician and neonatologist. The woman should be seen more frequently in pregnancy, to be screened for pre-eclampsia and IUGR. She should be screened for gestational diabetes if she is receiving steroid therapy. There should always be a high index of suspicion of relapse, even if symptoms seem compatible with normal pregnancy. She should receive the appropriate thromboprophylaxis treatment throughout pregnancy and the puerperium. Low-dose aspirin can be useful for the inhibition of inflammation, prevention of pre-eclampsia and thromboprophylaxis throughout pregnancy.

Postpartum haemorrhage has not been reported in association with Takayasu's arteritis. Intrapartum intravenous steroid support should be considered if the woman has been taking a dose of prednisolone equivalent to or greater than 7.5 mg/day in the 14 days preceding delivery.

Presence of untreated aneurysms might be an indication for operative delivery, especially if there has been a recent haemorrhage or for fetal salvage in the moribund mother.

5.20 PNEUMONIA

Mrs W was a 45 year old nonsmoking woman in her second pregnancy. Her first baby was delivered by Caesarean section at 37 weeks' gestation following a failed induction of labour for suspected fetal growth restriction.

She booked in the first trimester and had uncomplicated care with regular antenatal checks. Serial growth scans showed normal growth of the fetus on the 50th centile. Mrs W developed some shortness of breath at about 22 weeks' gestation, which subsequently resolved. At 32 weeks' gestation, it was noted that she had a productive cough.

At 34 weeks' gestation, Mrs W presented to the antenatal day unit with severe shortness of breath and a cough productive of green sputum. She had been unwell for more than 2 weeks and her cough had worsened over the past few days. The night before she had been unable to sleep because she was so dyspnoeic and she also had pleuritic chest pain radiating to the interscapular region. She was generally tired and exhausted. Mrs W was initially transferred to the delivery suite and then to the obstetric high-dependency unit when her clinical condition continued to deteriorate.

On examination, she was pyrexial, tachypnoeic, with a respiratory rate of 30/min, and using the accessory muscles of respiration. She could only talk in short sentences. Her blood pressure was 90/55 mmHg, her pulse was bounding at 130 bpm, the JVP was normal and auscultation of the heart revealed a soft ejection systolic murmur. There was decreased air entry and dullness to percussion at the left base, with coarse inspiratory and expiratory crackles. There was minimal ankle oedema. Blood gases that were performed while she was breathing air showed a pH of 7.469, a pCO_2 of 3.6 kPa, a pO_2 of 7.9 kPa and a base excess of -2.9. The differential diagnosis was of probable pneumonia and possible pulmonary embolism.

She was given facial oxygen at 3 l/min and clarithromycin, 500 mg intravenously twice daily and cefuroxime, 1.5 mg three times daily. A therapeutic dose of enoxaparin was also given to treat a possible pulmonary embolism. An urgent chest X-ray, echocardiogram and ECG were requested, the former confirming left lower lobe pneumonia. She was also given betamethasone for fetal lung maturation.

While Mrs W was being stabilized, the CTG showed recurrent variable decelerations. Repeat abdominal examination remained normal and there were no signs of an abruption. Blood gases were repeated 40 minutes later after she had received 10 l of oxygen, and the hypoxia had improved: pH, 7.459; pCO_2, 3.3 kPa; pO_2, 14 kPa; and base excess, -4.4. Mrs W remained unwell, and in the light of concerns for fetal well-being too, it was decided to stabilize and deliver her by urgent (grade 2) Caesarean section under a general anaesthetic. General anaesthesia was chosen because the recent therapeutic dose of enoxaparin precluded regional anaesthesia and, because of worsening maternal exhaustion, mechanical ventilation might become necessary.

The Caesarean section was uncomplicated, and a healthy nonacidotic, normally grown baby was delivered. Postpartum haemorrhage prophylaxis, in the form of a Syntocinon infusion, was started, because anaemia would potentially worsen Mrs W's oxygenation. Perioperatively Mrs X required noradrenaline (norepinephrine) and was transferred to the ICU for continued ventilation. Inotropic support was required for only a few hours.

The next day she was extubated without difficulty and transferred back to the obstetric high-dependency unit. Oxygen saturation was between 93% and 95% with air. Mrs W continued to improve over the next few days and her antibiotics were changed to oral preparations. On the fourth postoperative day, the oxygen saturation with room air was consistently >97%. The chest X-ray was repeated on day 9 and showed some bronchial thickening, but no residual consolidation. She went home the following day.

Discussion

Mrs W was unwell for some time and presented only once she became extremely sick; in hospital, she continued to deteriorate. She was resuscitated and stabilized, and delivered by Caesarean section for fetal distress.

Mrs W had two of the four BTS criteria for severe pneumonia and postoperatively required admission to ICU. Fortunately, she made a quick recovery, with minimal morbidity.

Pregnant women do not get pneumonia more often than nonpregnant women, but it can result in greater morbidity and mortality because of the physiological adaptations of pregnancy [69]. The hormonal effects of progesterone and beta-human chorionic gonadotrophins, changes in chest dimension and elevation of the diaphragm all result in a state of relative dyspnoea, which worsens in the third trimester. Changes in maternal oxygen consumption and tidal volume result in a decreased capacity to compensate for respiratory disease.

Additionally, pregnancy results in a compensated respiratory alkalosis. Minute ventilation increases, in addition to the increase in pO_2 to 13–14 kPa (104–108 mmHg), whereas pCO_2 decreases to 4.0 kPa (30; 27–32 mmHg). The arterial pH is maintained through increased renal excretion of bicarbonate. Small changes in these compensated values can indicate more severe respiratory dysfunction than outside pregnancy and can alter fetal oxygenation. Co-existing maternal disease, such as asthma and anaemia, increase the risk of pneumonia in pregnancy. Neonatal consequences include low birth weight and premature delivery in 44% of patients.

The estimated prevalence of antepartum pneumonia ranges from 0.78 in 1000 to 2.7 in 1000 deliveries. Pregnancy increases the risk of maternal complications from community-acquired pneumonia, such as mechanical ventilation (10–20%), bacteraemia (16%) and empyema (8%). The advent of antibiotics has reduced maternal mortality from 23% to <4%.

The most common organisms implicated in community-acquired pneumonia are *Streptococcus pneumonia, Haemophilus influenza* and *Mycoplasma pneumonia* [70]. Viral pneumonia contributes 5% of the pathogens, the commonest being influenza and varicella. Clinical symptoms include fever, cough (59%), pleuritic chest pain (27%), rigors and dyspnoea (32%) [71]. On examination, there is usually tachypnoea, dullness to percussion, vocal fremitus and use of the accessory muscles. Auscultation could reveal a pleural friction rub, inspiratory rales or absent breath sounds. Because physical examination is only 47–69% sensitive and 58–75% specific, all cases must be confirmed by chest X-ray [72]. Of patients with pneumonia, 98% have abnormal chest X-rays. The differential diagnosis should include pulmonary embolism, cholecystitis, appendicitis and pyelonephritis.

The optimal location for treatment (e.g. as an out-patient or in-patient, or in the ICU) can be decided by using the BTS guidelines [73]: consider that the presence of two or more of the following four criteria indicates severe disease:

Respiratory rate of >30 breaths/min
Diastolic blood pressure of <60 mmHg
Blood urea nitrogen of >19.1 mg/dl
Confusion

The pregnancy-associated fall in blood pressure means that the second criterion might not necessarily indicate circulatory compromise.

Patients with two or more of the above criteria are considered to have severe disease, and have a 36-fold increase in mortality: they are candidates for elective admission to the ICU. Management of pneumonia in pregnancy includes admission, initiation of antimicrobial therapy, evaluation of fetal well-being and maintenance of normal maternal respiratory function. Supplemental oxygen is required in the majority of patients to treat the increased alveolar–arterial oxygenation gradient. Any reversible airway obstruction should be treated and physiotherapy is advisable.

ICU admission and intubation are indicated if there is inadequate ventilation, a need for airway protection or persistent metabolic acidosis. Although elective delivery has been advocated to improve maternal respiratory status, there is little evidence to support this. Several authors have concluded that delivery should be performed only for obstetric indications.

In the case of Mrs W, delivery was indicated for fetal indications but was delayed until the maternal condition had stabilized enough to proceed with anaesthesia and surgery.

5.21 TYPE IV EHLERS-DANLOS SYNDROME: TWO MANAGEMENT DILEMMAS

Ms Y, a 28 year old nulliparous woman, attended for prepregnancy counselling. She gave a history of type IV (vascular) Ehlers-Danlos syndrome (EDS). She was in a long-term relationship and had been considering a pregnancy for some time. She was using condoms for contraception and had never previously been pregnant.

In her personal history, she had had recurrent shoulder dislocations and had frequently attended the accident and emergency department. The possibility of a stabilizing operation on the shoulder joint had been discussed by the orthopaedic surgeons.

She reported easy bleeding from her gums. An echocardiogram, performed because of a heart murmur, showed mild mitral regurgitation only. She had deliberately not investigated the significance of EDS either in pregnancy or outside pregnancy because she "did not want to be frightened" by the information.

In her family history, her mother, who has EDS, had a history of a DVT in her 30 s and had had two pregnancies ending in two normal deliveries. She had one younger sister, with a history of easy bruising and bleeding, who had died suddenly 3 years previously at the age of 25 years. A postmortem gave "natural causes" as the cause of death.

Mrs X, a 30 year old Caucasian woman was referred to the obstetric medicine clinic at 16 weeks' gestation for discussion regarding her possible diagnosis of type IV EDS. She was first suspected to have this condition 1 year previously when she presented with a spontaneous pneumothorax. Following recovery from this, a tissue biopsy was planned, but she conceived and it was therefore deferred. In her family history, her sister, who was known to have type IV EDS, died at the age of 21 years from an aortic rupture, having previously had an aortic-root replacement.

She had had four successful pregnancies in the past, before the pneumothorax. The first ended with an uncomplicated Caesarean section after failed induction of labour for prolonged pregnancy; postoperative convalescence was normal. She then had three successful VBACs, the last two births taking <4 hours. There were no associated traumatic or haemorrhagic complications in any of the deliveries. There was no history of prolonged bleeding or easy bruising at any time.

On examination, she did not exhibit skin hyperelasticity or joint hypermobility. However, she did have the characteristic circinate rash on the medial aspect of one foot. Examination of the respiratory and cardiovascular systems was normal. Her prepregnancy echocardiogram was normal.

On balance, it was felt that there was a high chance that she had type IV EDS, and termination of pregnancy was discussed with her. She decided to continue with the pregnancy, acknowledging the 25% mortality risk, because she felt reassured by her previously successful confinements. She was kept under close surveillance by an obstetrician and an obstetric physician.

An echocardiogram performed in pregnancy revealed normal chambers and large vessels. There were trivial mitral, tricuspid and aortic valve prolapses. A fetal anomaly scan was normal. The following care plan was made:

Await spontaneous labour.

Aim for spontaneous vaginal delivery.

Elective admission at 38 weeks' gestation (because she lived far from the tertiary centre).

Planned early epidural anaesthesia in labour.

Normal intrapartum and postpartum monitoring and management.

Intravenous access in labour.

Active management of the third stage of labour.

Shortened second stage of labour.

If Caesarean section is required, the following steps will be necessary:

(a) A senior obstetrician must be present for the operation.

(b) A polydioxanone surgical (non-absorbable) (PDS) suture must be used to close the rectus sheath.

Nonabsorbable material must be used for skin closure.
Antibiotic cover for 48 hours.

Subsequent obstetric events were uneventful. She had a normal anomaly scan at 20 weeks' gestation, with a normal uterine artery Doppler study. She was admitted at 38 weeks' gestation, as planned. After 1 week, she was increasingly distressed by being separated from her family. Her cervix was favourable, and so an amniotomy was performed to induce labour. She delivered a healthy infant, exhibiting no signs of EDS.

Discussion

EDS is a spectrum of conditions characterized by defect either in the synthesis or in the structure of connective tissue. There are 10 variants of EDS, types I–X. It is often difficult to assign patients to a specific classification because the biochemical and clinical criteria are difficult to define. Furthermore, people with the milder form of the disease have no need to seek medical advice. Thus, it is difficult to ascertain the true incidence and definition of the spectrum of EDS. It is estimated that EDS occurs in approximately 1 in 5000 individuals. It is more common in black people.

From a clinical and obstetric point of view, type I and type IV EDS are the most relevant and carry the most morbidity. Type I EDS is the classic form of the disease, characterized by hypermobility of the joints and hyperelasticity of the skin, which is prone to "cigarette paper burns".

Type IV EDS, also known as the "ecchymotic" or "vascular" form, is generally inherited as an autosomal dominant condition. Type IV EDS causes severe fragility of connective tissues and is associated with sudden death from arterial and visceral rupture and complications of surgical and radiological interventions. Vessels commonly affected include the iliac, splenic and renal arteries and the aorta. This results in either massive haematoma or death. Repeated rupture of viscera and diverticulae could be the presenting symptoms.

Hypermobility of large joints, characteristic of other types of EDS, is an uncommon finding in patients with vascular EDS, but recurrent shoulder dislocations occur (as in Ms Y). In contrast to type I EDS, skin changes are more prominent in type IV EDS. The basic defect lies in the synthesis or structure of type III procollagen, which is found abundantly in viscera, vessels and the uterus. Delay in diagnosis is common, and in adulthood, four main clinical findings – a striking facial appearance, easy bruising, translucent skin with visible veins and rupture of vessels and gravid uterus or intestines – contribute to the diagnosis. Arterial rupture and intestinal perforation develop in

25% of patients before the age of 20 years and 80% of patients before the age of 40 years. In a recent series, the median survival was 48 years.

A search of the literature relating to pregnancy was performed, in order to advise Ms Y and Mrs X. The world literature reports fewer than 200 cases of type IV EDS in pregnancy. Complications of EDS are more common in pregnancy. Obstetric complications include prelabour rupture of membranes, preterm labour, precipitate labour, abnormal lie of an affected fetus, antepartum haemorrhage, postpartum haemorrhage from perineal trauma and uterine rupture. The risk of mortality is highest, from vascular rupture, during the antenatal period and the initial 2 weeks postpartum. Although mortality rates as high as 25% have been quoted, a more recent review quotes 6% [74,75].

The largest series reports 183 pregnancies in 81 cases [76]. There were 167 deliveries of live born infants at term, three stillbirths, 10 spontaneous abortions and three voluntary terminations. There were 12 deaths in the peripartum period: five deaths from uterine rupture during labour, two deaths from vessel rupture at delivery, and five deaths in the postpartum period after vessel rupture. The incidence of preterm delivery was reported as 12.4%.

Before this series, the largest case series was published in 1983 [77]. This paper describes 10 women who had had 20 pregnancies; five women had died as a result of pregnancy-related complications. The overall risk of death in each pregnancy within this group was 25%. In this paper, two cases are described in detail, one case in which the woman was admitted at 28 weeks' gestation in preterm labour (with EDS undiagnosed). As labour progressed, she suddenly collapsed and was unable to be resuscitated. At postmortem, she was found to have a ruptured thoracic aorta in two places between which a dissection had occurred. There was also a tear in the uterus. In the second case, the woman presented in her third pregnancy in labour at term. During the second stage of labour, the contractions stopped and the fetal heart could not be heard. An emergency Caesarean section was performed and she was found to have a ruptured uterus. Surgical repair was attempted but haemostasis could not be achieved and the patient died. The baby also died.

The morbidity rate could be as high as 25%. Surgical complications include arterial bleeding, easy tissue shearing, trauma resulting in further haemorrhage, infection and delayed healing. The two most common forms of congenital abnormality among infants born to mothers with EDS are talipes and congenital dislocation of the hip.

Ms Y was counselled that pregnancy would be associated with a significant risk of maternal death (10–15%). The main risk seems to be peripartum, but there is no evidence that elective delivery by

Caesarean section reduces the risk of arterial rupture, in particular. She specifically asked about the risks of termination of pregnancy if she became pregnant and the child was found to be affected. This would be a lesser risk than a pregnancy going to full term. However, because she would be pregnant for at least 12 weeks to enable prenatal diagnosis and termination, this would be an increased risk compared with not becoming pregnant. (One published case reports an intestinal rupture at 8 weeks' gestation [77].)

Because it was very important that Ms Y did not have an unplanned pregnancy, contraception was discussed. The progesterone-only pill, Implanon or the Mirena IUS, would be suitable and effective methods to use. Ms Y was made aware of the need to contact the obstetric medicine clinic should she become pregnant and was informed that she would be fully supported if she decided to go ahead with a pregnancy.

The dilemma in managing Mrs X included the lack of a precise diagnosis in a potentially lethal condition, causing anxiety to the clinicians caring for her. Although there were some features of the history and signs suggestive of the disease, there were negative factors as well. She had had an uncomplicated Caesarean section in the past, with no evidence of haemorrhage, postoperative infection or bleeding. This was followed by three successful VBACs, when one might have expected scar and even spontaneous uterine rupture to complicate delivery. These vaginal births were not associated with bleeding or trauma. All her children seem well, although none had yet been tested. In addition, it is known that the risk of complications from type IV EDS increases with age. Hence, Mrs X might have been "relatively" protected in her past pregnancies and birthing experiences and more at risk in her current pregnancy. The possibility was significant and the consequences potentially lethal, hence the option of termination of pregnancy when she presented at 16 weeks' gestation. It has been suggested that EDS is associated with IUGR, but these claims have originated from case reports. Serial growth ultrasound scans were not performed for this lady because her uterine artery Doppler study was normal and her past obstetric history did not suggest increased risk of IUGR.

5.22 SUPRAVENTRICULAR TACHYCARDIA

Mrs Z, a fit and healthy 40 year old lady of African origin whose two previous pregnancies were uncomplicated, experienced episodes of palpitations from the 16th week of her current pregnancy. These episodes lasted 4–5 hours and occurred approximately three times weekly. At 21 weeks' gestation, during an episode of palpitations, she had a syncopal attack. At 23 weeks' gestation, she had a second syncopal episode, and presented to the emergency unit. On both occasions, her 12-lead ECG was normal, simply showing sinus tachycardia.

She was a nonsmoker, with no personal or family history of cardiac disease. There was no history of rheumatic fever.

On examination, her blood pressure was normal and her pulse was 90 bpm and regular. Examination of the cardiovascular system was normal. The 12-lead ECG was normal, with no evidence of ischaemia or arrhythmia; there were no delta waves in the precordial leads. Echocardiography was normal.

A 24-hour ambulatory ECG (Holter monitoring) showed paroxysmal supraventricular tachycardia (SVT) with runs as high as 200 bpm, which co-incided with her feeling faint. There were also runs of bradycardia suggestive of type I heart block.

Oral flecainide therapy, 50 mg twice daily was commenced, with a dramatic resolution of symptoms. Therapy was continued throughout pregnancy and postpartum. Fetal echocardiography was normal.

The pregnancy progressed normally to 36 weeks' gestation, when she developed severe pre-eclampsia that required urgent delivery by Caesarean section, which was complicated by massive postpartum haemorrhage of 2000 ml of blood.

She underwent slow pathway ablation for atrioventricular (AV) nodal re-entry tachycardia 3 months postpartum, which proved successful. Flecainide was discontinued.

Discussion

Cardiac arrhythmias can occur in a heart that appears structurally normal or originate from scar tissue due to structural disease, including, for example, abnormal heart valves, scarring secondary to surgical correction of congenital heart disease and coronary artery disease. In some cases, there might be a genetic predisposition. Pregnancy can increase the incidence of palpitations, possibly because of the normal tachycardia of pregnancy, increased re-entry phenomena, the anterior rotation of the heart and hyperdynamic circulation of pregnancy increasing the sensation of an abnormal heart beat or a lower threshold and greater opportunity for presenting with palpitations to health carers; the evidence for this comes from small case series and anecdote. In a large survey conducted over 2 years and involving 107 subjects, it was noted that the risk of having a first episode of tachyarrhythmia was 3.9%, which was thought to be similar to the background rate. However, if the subjects were pregnant at diagnosis, they were at a 22% increased risk of having more severe or frequent attacks [78].

The most common arrhythmias encountered in pregnancy are SVTs, atrial premature contractions (APCs) and ventricular premature contractions (VPCs) [79]. These are usually not sustained, and resolve spontaneously. Of pregnant women aged over 40 years who had "routine" Holter monitoring, 60% had some form of arrhythmia [80], the majority of which were asymptomatic. Sustained arrhythmia is rare, occurring in 2–3 out of 1000 pregnancies [81].

The predominant symptoms of arrhythmia are palpitations, dizziness, syncope and sudden death. Palpitations are a relatively common symptom of pregnancy, and it can be very difficult to differentiate physiology from pathology in the pregnant setting. In one study, only 10% of symptomatic patients were diagnosed with arrhythmia [82]. Ultimately, the decision to investigate further depends on the severity of symptoms, presence of risk factors and physical signs. A 12-lead ECG is usually only diagnostic if performed during a palpitation. However, it could indicate other relevant information, such as the presence of a structural abnormality, coronary artery disease or delta waves (suggesting Wolff–Parkinson–White syndrome). The definitive tests for paroxysmal arrhythmias are 24-hour Holter monitoring or event monitoring.

The primary treatment for acute SVT remains vagal stimulation, including self-administered carotid massage, Valsalva manoeuvre, bulbar pressure or ice-cold water wipes over the face. Primary treatment is only effective in 50% of cases, and medical therapy should be considered in those who do not respond, especially if symptoms are sustained or severe. Adenosine, an endogenous nucleoside, is ultra-short-acting, with a plasma half-life of <2 seconds. It is safe and effective in pregnancy, but should be avoided in women with asthma because it could precipitate bronchospasm. Propranolol and verapamil are also used for terminating SVTs. There are no data that directly compare these agents, but verapamil has had adverse effects reported, including fetal death, and should not be the agent of first choice. There is increasing experience of flecainide use in the treatment of arrhythmias, especially in Wolff–Parkinson–White syndrome. This is largely because it is the drug of choice for the in-utero treatment of fetal SVTs, for which it has been shown to be superior to digoxin [83]. It is considered to be safe in pregnancy, although it is still classified as a category C drug by the FDA. In Mrs Z, flecainide was preferred to beta-blockers such as sotalol because there was a concern that the latter might worsen the episodes of bradycardia. In resistant cases DC, cardioversion is an option, which is considered to be safe in pregnancy [84] with no known adverse effects on the mother or fetus. If symptomatic attacks are frequent, prophylaxis should be considered.

Ultimately, the definitive treatment is to eliminate the cause of the attacks. Electrophysiological conduction studies can be performed in pregnancy to detect and treat aberrant conducting pathways, and this should be considered if medical therapy fails.

REFERENCES

1. Nelson-Piercy C. Haematological problems. In: *Handbook of Obstetric Medicine*, 3rd edn. Informa Healthcare, London; 2006: 277–81.
2. Letsky E. Anaemia. In: James KD, Steer PJ, Weiner CP and Gonik B (eds) *High Risk Pregnancy Management Options*, 2nd edn. WB Saunders, London; 1999: 729–65.
3. Liggins GC. The treatment of missed abortion by high dosage syntocinon intravenous infusion. *J Obst Gynaecol Br Empire* 1962; **69**: 277–81.
4. Eggers TR and Fliegner JR. Water Intoxication and Syntocinon Infusion. *Aust NZ J Obstet Gynaecol* 1979; **19**: 59–60.
5. Mackenzie IZ. Labour induction including pregnancy, termination for fetal anomaly. In: James KD, Steer PJ, Weiner CP and Gonik B (eds) *High Risk Pregnancy Management Options*, 2nd edn. WB Saunders, London; 1999: 1091.
6. Stratton JF et al. Hyponatraemia and non electrolytic solutions in labouring patients. *Eur J Obstet Gynaecol Reprod Biol* 1995; **59**: 149–51.
7. Chappell LC et al. Effect of antioxidants on the occurrence of pre-eclampsia in women at increased risk: a randomised trial. *Lancet* 1999; **354**: 810–6.
8. Hankins GD et al. Myocardial infarction during pregnancy: a review. *Obstet Gynecol* 1985; **65**: 139–46.
9. Roth A and Elkayam U. Acute myocardial infarction associated with pregnancy. *Ann Intern Med* 1996; **125**: 751–62.
10. Quan A. Fetopathy associated with exposure to angiotensin converting enzyme inhibitors and angiotensin receptor antagonists. *Early Hum Dev* 2006; **82**: 23–8.
11. Diav-Citrin O et al. The safety of proton pump inhibitors in pregnancy: a multicentre prospective controlled study. *Aliment Pharmacol Ther* 2005; **21**: 269–75.
12. Nishiguchi T and Kobayashi T. Antiphospholipid syndrome: characteristics and obstetrical management. *Current Drug Targets* 2005; **6**: 593–605.
13. Baxi LV and Rho RB. Pregnancy after Cardiac Transplantation. *Am J Obstet Gynecol* 1993; **169**: 33–34.

14. Morini A et al. Pregnancy after heart transplant: update and case report. *Human Reprod* 1998; **13**: 749–57.
15. Branch KR et al. Risks of subsequent pregnancies on mother and newborn in female heart transplant recipients. *J Heart Lung Transplant* 1998; **17**: 698–702.
16. Chames MC and Livingston JC. Late post partum eclampsia: A preventable disease? *Am J Obstet Gynecol* 2002; **186**: 1174–7.
17. Dziewas R and Stogbauer F. Late onset post partum eclampsia: a rare and difficult diagnosis. *J Neurol* 2002; **249**: 1287–91.
18. Isler CM and Barrilleaux PS. Repeat post partum magnesium sulfate administration for convulsion prophylaxis: is there a patient profile predictive of need for additional therapy? *J Maternal Fetal Neonatal Med* 2002; **11**: 75–9.
19. Ogunyemi DA, Michelini GA (2006). Hyperemesis gravidarum. http://www. emedicine.com/med/topic 1075.htm (accessed 12/07/2006).
20. Goodwin TM et al. Transient hyperthyroidism and hyperemesis gravidarum: clinical aspects. *Am J Obstet Gynecol* 1992; **167**: 648–52.
21. Bagis T et al. Endoscopy in hyperemesis gravidarum and Helicobacter pylori infection. *Int J Gynaecol Obstet* 2002; **79**: 105–9.
22. Nelson-Piercy C et al. Randomized, placebo-controlled trial of corticosteroids for hyperemesis gravidarum. *Br J Obset Gynaecol* 2001; **108**: 1–7.
23. Moran P and Taylor R. Management of hyperemesis gravidarum: the importance of weight loss as a criterion for steroid therapy. *QJM* 2002; **95**: 153–8.
24. Pathan M and Kittner SJ. Pregnancy and Stroke. *Curr Neurol Neurosci Rep* 2003; **3**: 27–31.
25. Hildebrandt R et al. Hypokalaemia in pregnant women treated with beta 2-mimetic drug fenoterol. *J Perinat Med* 1997; **25**: 173–9.
26. Damallie KK et al. Hypokalaemic periodic paralysis in pregnancy after 1-hour glucose screen. *Obstet Gynecol* 2000; **95**: 1037.
27. Appel CC et al. Caffeine-induced hypokalemic paralysis in pregnancy. *Obstet Gynecol* 2001; **97**: 805–7.
28. Matsunami K et al. Hypokalemia in a pregnant woman with heavy cola consumption. *Int J Obstet Gynaecol* 1994; **44**: 283–4.
29. Ukaonu C et al. Hypokalaemia myopathy in pregnancy caused by clay ingestion. *Obstet Gynecol* 2003; **102**: 1169–71.
30. Hardardottir H et al. Renal tubular acidosis in pregnancy: case report and literature review. *J Mat-Fet Med* 1997; **6**: 16–20.
31. Duff P. Hepatitis in pregnancy. *Semin Perinatol* 1998; **22**: 277–83.

32. Knox TA and Olan LB. Current concepts: Liver disease in pregnancy. *N Engl J Med* 1996; **335**: 569–76.
33. Moosa M and Mazzaferri EL. Outcome of differentiated thyroid cancer diagnosed in pregnant women. *J Clin Endocrinol Metab* 1997; **82**: 2862–6.
34. Chloe W and McDougall IR. Thyroid cancer in pregnant women: Diagnostic and therapeutic management. *Thyroid* 1994; **4**: 4333–435.
35. O'Doherty MJ et al. Treating thyrotoxicosis in pregnant or potentially pregnant women: The risk to the fetus is very low. *Br Med J* 1999; **318**: 5–6.
36. Guidelines for Management Thyroid Cancer in Adults British Thyroid Association and Royal College Physicians (2002). http://www.british-thyroid-association.org.uk (accessed November 2004)
37. Eichinger S. D-dimer testing in pregnancy. *Semin Vasc Med* 2005; **5**: 375–8.
38. Scarsbrook AF et al. Diagnosis of suspected venous thromboembolic disease in pregnancy. *Clin Radiol* 2006; **61**: 1–12.
39. Ray JG and WS Chan. Deep Vein Thrombosis During Pregnancy and the Puerperium: A Meta-Analysis of the Period of Risk and the Leg of Presentation. *Obstet Gynecol* 1999; **54**: 265–71.
40. RCOG green top guideline. Clinical Green Top Guidelines. Thromboembolic Disease in Pregnancy and the Puerperium: Acute Management (28) – Apr 2001 http://www.rcog.org.uk/index.asp? page ID=533.
41. Ayoub C et al. The pregnant cardiac woman (Obstetric and gynaecological anaesthesia). *Curr Opin Anaesthesiol* 2002; **15**: 285–91.
42. Nelson-Piercy C. Heart disease. In: *Handbook of Obstetric Medicine*, 3rd edn. Informa Healthcare, London; 2006: 23–43.
43. Lupton M et al. Cardiac disease in pregnancy. *Curr Opin Obstet Gynaecol* 2002; **14**: 137–43.
44. Henry M et al. BTS guidelines for the management of spontaneous pneumothorax. *Thorax* 2003; **58(suppl. II)**: ii39–ii52.
45. Baumann MH et al. Management of spontaneous pneumothorax: An American College of Chest Physicians Delphi Consensus Statement. *Chest* 2001; **119**: 590–602.
46. Baumann MH. Treatment of spontaneous pneumothorax. *Curr Opin Pulm Med* 2000; **6**: 275–80.
47. Diethelm L. Diagnostic imaging of the lung during pregnancy. *Clin Obstet Gynecol* 1996; **39**: 36–55.
48. Yim APC. Thoracoscopy in the management of pneumothorax. *Curr Opin Pulm Med* 2001; **7**: 210–14.

49. Richards A et al. The genetics and pathogenesis of haemolytic uraemic syndrome and thrombotic thrombocytopaenic purpura. *Curr Opin Nephrol Hypertens* 2002; **11:** 431–5.
50. Yarranton H and Machin S. An update on the pathogenesis and management of acquired thrombotic thrombocytopaenic purpura. *Curr Opin Neurol* 2003; **16:** 367–73.
51. Bastani B et al. Cyclosporine-associated post-partum haemolytic uraemic syndrome in a renal transplant patient: lack of response to plasmapheresis but remission after intravenous immunoglobulin G. *Nephrology* 2001; **6:** 133–7.
52. Roberts G et al. Acute renal failure complicating HELLP syndrome, SLE and anti-phospholipid syndrome: Successful outcome using plasma exchange therapy. *Lupus* 2003; **12:** 251–7.
53. Kumar P and Clark M (eds). Haematological disease. In: *Kumar and Clark Clinical Medicine,* 5th edn. WB Saunders, Edinburgh; 2002: 405–72.
54. Carr JA et al. Surgical indications in idiopathic splenomegaly. *Arch Surgery* 2002; **137:** 64–8.
55. George JN and Vesely SK. Immune thrombocytopenic purpura – Let the treatment fit the patient. *New Engl J Med* 2003; **349:** 903–5.
56. Kam PCA et al. Thrombocytopenia in the parturient. *Anaesthesia* 2004; **59:** 255–64.
57. Rietberg CC and Lindhout D. Adult patients with spina bifida cystica: genetic counselling, pregnancy and delivery. *Eur J Obstet Gynecol Reprod Biol* 1993; **52:** 63–70.
58. Arata M et al. Pregnancy outcome and complications in women with spina bifida. *J Reprod Med* 2000; **45:** 743–8.
59. To WW and Wong MW. Kyphoscoliosis complicating pregnancy. *Int J Gynaecol Obstet* 1996; **55:** 123–8.
60. Restrick LJ et al. Nasal ventilation in pregnancy: treatment of nocturnal hypoventilation in a patient with kyphoscoliosis. *Eur Resp J* 1997; **10:** 2657–8.
61. Jenkins RE et al. Pemphigoid Gestationis. *Br J Dermatol* 1995; **49:** 595–8.
62. Freiman A and Pabby A (2006). Pemphigoid Gestationis. http://www.emedicine.com/derm/topic178.htm (accessed October 2006)
63. Kennedy CTC and Kyle P. Skin disease. In: James KD, Steer PJ, Weiner CP and Gonik B (eds) *High Risk Pregnancy Management Options,* 2nd edn. WB Saunders, London; 1999: 921–2.
64. Nelson-Piercy C. Skin disease. In: *Handbook of Obstetric Medicine,* 3rd edn. Informa Healthcare, London; 2006: 263–71.
65. Kerr GS et al. Takayasu's Arteritis. *Ann Int Med* 1994; **120:** 919–29.

66. Johnston SL et al. Takayasu arteritis: a review. *J Clin Path* 2002; **55:** 481–86.
67. Sun Y et al. Ultrasonographic study and long term follow-up of patients with Takayasu's Arteritis. *Stroke* 1996; **27:** 2178–82.
68. Mwipate BP et al. Takayasu arteritis: clinical features and management: report of 272 cases. *ANZ J Surgery* 2005; **75:** 110–17.
69. Jenkins TM et al. *Am J Obstet Gynecol* 1989; **161:** 657–62.
70. Lim WS et al. Treatment of community-acquired lower respiratory tract infections during pregnancy. *Am J Respir Med* 2003; **2:** 221–33.
71. Munn MB et al. Pneumonia as a complication of pregnancy. *J Matern Fetal Med* 1999; **8:** 151–4.
72. Kasper DL et al. (eds) *Harrison's Principles of Internal Medicine*, 16th edn. McGraw-Hill, New York; 2005.
73. British Thoracic Society Pneumonia Guideline Committee. Guideline for the management of community acquired pneumonia in adults. *Thorax* 2001; 56(suppl IV): 1–64.
74. Lind J and Wallenburg HC. Pregnancy and the Ehlers-Danlos syndrome. *Acta Obstet Gynecol Scand* 2002; **81:** 293–300.
75. Campbell N and Rosaeg OP. Anaesthetic management of a parturient with Ehlers Danlos syndrome type IV. *Can J Anaesth* 2002; **49:** 493–6.
76. Pepin M et al. Clinical and genetic features of Ehlers-Danlos Syndrome Type IV, the Vascular type. *New Engl J Med* 2000; **342:** 673–80.
77. Rudd NL and Holbrook KA. Pregnancy complications in Type IV Ehlers-Danlos syndrome. *Lancet* 1983; **321:** 249–50.
78. Lee SH et al. Effects of pregnancy on first onset and symptoms of paroxysmal supraventricular tachycardia. *Am J Cardiol* 1995; *76:* 675–8.
79. Nelson-Piercy C. Heart disease in pregnancy. *Acta Anaesth Belg* 2002; **53:** 321–6.
80. Hunter S and Robson SC. Adaptation of the maternal heart in pregnancy. *Br Heart J* 1992; **68:** 540–3.
81. Blomstrom-Lundqvist C et al. ACC/AHA/ESC guidelines for the management of patients with supraventricular arrhythmias – executive summary: a report of the American College of Cardiology/American Heart Association Task Force on Practice Guidelines and the European Society of Cardiology Committee for Practice Guidelines (Writing Committee to Develop Guidelines for the Management of Patients With Supraventricular Arrhythmias). *Circulation* 2003; **108:** 1871–909.

82. Shotan A et al. Incidence of Arrhythmias in normal pregnancy and relationship to palpitations, dizziness and syncope. *Am J Obstet Gynecol* 1997; **79:** 1061–4.

83. Jaglar J and Page R. Antiarrhythmic drugs in pregnancy. *Curr Opin Cardiol* 2001; **16:** 40–5.

84. Finlay AY and Edmunds V. DC cardioversion in pregnancy. *Br J Clin Pract* 1979; **33:** 88–94.

Glossary

ACE: angiotensin converting enzyme
ACTH: adrenocorticotrophic hormone
ADH: antidiuretic hormone
AFLP: acute fatty liver of pregnancy
AIHA: autoimmune haemolytic anaemia
AlkP: alkaline phosphatase
ALT: alanine transaminase
ARM: artificial rupture of membranes
AST: aspartate transaminase
AP: anteroposterior
APS: antiphospholipid syndrome
AV: atrioventricular
CEMACH: Confidential Enquiry into Maternal and Child Health
Cl^-: chloride
Cr: creatinine
CRP: C reactive protein
CT: computerised tomography
CTG: cardiotocograph
CVS: chorionic villus sampling
DAU: Day Assessment Unit
DC: direct current
DEXA: dual energy X ray absorptiometry
DI: diabetes insipidus
DIC: disseminated intravascular coagulopathy
DVT: deep vein thrombosis
ECG: electrocardiogram
EFW: estimated fetal weight
ESR: erythrocyte sedimentation rate
FBC: full blood count
FEV_1: forced expiratory volume in one second
fT_4: free thyroxine
FSH: follicle stimulating hormone
FVC: forced vital capacity

Gamma GT: gamma glutamyl transpeptidase
GH: growth hormone
HbA_{1c}: glycosylated haemoglobin
Hb: haemoglobin
HCO_3^-: bicarbonate
HCG: human chorionic gonadotrophin
HELLP: haemolysis, elevated liver enzymes and low platelets
HG: hyperemesis gravidarum
HIT: heparin induced thrombocytopenia
HIV: human immunodeficiency virus
HUS: haemolytic uraemic syndrome
INR: international normalised ratio
ITP: idiopathic thrombocytopenic purpura
IUGR: intrauterine growth restriction
JVP: jugular venous pressure
K^+: potassium
LFT: liver function tests
LH: luteinising hormone
LMWH: low molecular weight heparin
LSCS: lower segment Caesarean section
MCHC: mean cell haemoglobin concentration
MCV: mean cell volume
$MgSO_4$: magnesium sulphate
MRI: magnetic resonance imaging
MSU: mid stream urine
Na^+: sodium
NASH: non-alcoholic steatohepatitis
NSAIDS: non steroidal anti-inflammatory drugs
NTD: neural tube defect
OC: obstetric cholestasis
OCP: combined oral contraceptive pill
PA: posterior: anterior
pCO_2: partial pressure of carbon dioxide
PET: pre-eclampsia
PHT: pulmonary hypertension
PKU: phenyl ketonuria
pO_2: partial pressure of oxygen
POP: progestogen only pill
PSC: primary sclerosing cholangitis
PTU: propylthiouracil
PV: per vaginam
RBG: random blood glucose
RCOG: Royal College of Obstetricians and Gynaecologists
RCP: Royal College of Physicians

RNA: ribonucleic acid
SLE: systemic lupus erythematosus
SVT: supraventricular tachycardia
TB: tuberculosis
TSH: thyroid stimulating hormone
TTP: thrombocytopenic purpura
U: urea
UC: ulcerative colitis
UDCA: ursodeoxycholic acid
UH: unfractionated heparin
VBAC: vaginal birth after Caesarean section
VSD: ventricular septal defect
VZIG: varicella zoster immunoglobulin
WBC: white blood cell

Index

Lightning Source UK Ltd.
Milton Keynes UK
UKHW04f0209210818
327417UK00001BA/19/P